Review of Research in Nursing Education

William L. Holzemer, Ph.D.

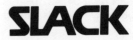

William L. Holzemer, Ph.D., Editor

Associate Professor
  Department of Physiological Nursing

Coordinator
  Program Research and Development

Office of Academic Programs

School of Nursing

University of California, San Francisco

Contents

Part One: Nursing Education in the Academic Setting

Part Two: Nursing Education in the Service Setting

Contributors

June Bailey, R.N., Ed.D., F.A.A.N.
Professor and Associate Dean
School of Nursing
University of California, San Francisco
San Francisco, California

Pamela Baj, R.N., M.S.
Assistant Professor
School of Nursing
University of San Francisco
San Francisco, California

Lillian A. Bargagliotti, R.N., M.S.N.
Assistant Professor
School of Nursing
Ohlone College
Fremont, California

Bette Case, R.N., M.S.N.
Administrative Coordinator
Academic Affiliation
Michael Reese Hospital
Chicago, Illinois

Richard E. Grant, R.N., Ph.D.
Assistant Professor
School of Nursing
University of Arizona
Tempe, Arizona

William L. Holzemer, Ph.D.
Associate Professor
School of Nursing
University of California, San Francisco
San Francisco, California

Deborah Marks, R.N., M.P.H.
Administrative Coordinator of Continuing Education
Michael Reese Hospital
Chicago, Illinois

Mary O'Leary, R.N., M.H.P.Ed.
Director of Education, Staff Development, and Research
Michael Reese Hospital
Chicago, Illinois

CONTRIBUTORS (cont.)

Elizabeth J. Pugh, R.N., Ph.D.
Associate Chairperson and Associate Professor
Department of Pediatric Nursing
Rush University
Rush-Presbyterian-St. Luke's Medical Center
Chicago, Illinois

Patricia Sparacino, R.N., M.S.
Assistant Clinical Professor
University of California, San Francisco
San Francisco, California

Christine A. Tanner, R.N., Ph.D.
Associate Professor, Graduate Studies Department,
   School of Nursing
University of Oregon, Health Sciences Center
Portland, Oregon

Annita B. Watson, R.N., D.N.S.
Professor and Chairperson
Division of Nursing
Sacramento State University
Sacramento, California

Preface

The purpose of this review text is to provide an analytical review and synthesis of research that has been conducted in nursing education. The volume is designed to assist the nursing educator in the academic and service arena. It is anticipated that it will serve as a resource for reviewing work accomplished to date for program planning. Also, researchers in these areas may utilize these reviews to assist them in planning further work. Topics are selected in areas where there has been sufficient research to allow a review to be conducted.

The text is organized in two parts. Part One reviews five topics of interest to nursing educators in the academic setting. These include research on clinical judgment, professional socialization, clinical teaching, predictors of academic success, and stress and the R.N. student. Part Two reviews three topics of interest to the nursing educator in the service setting. These include stress and critical care nursing, hospital staff development, and the clinical nurse specialist.

Future volumes will address additional topics of interest to nursing educators. If you wish to submit a topic for consideration for the review series, please write to the editor.

PART ONE: NURSING EDUCATION IN THE ACADEMIC SETTING

Chapter One:
Research on Clinical Judgment

Chapter One:
Research on Clinical Judgment

Christine A. Tanner, R.N., Ph.D.

A major goal in the education of virtually all health professionals is to enable students to make sound clinical judgments. In nursing, the specific instructional objectives related to clinical judgment are contained within the framework of the nursing process — a linear sequence of thought processes which includes the steps of assessment, planning, intervention and evaluation. Instructional methods to achieve these objectives are few. As a result, those of us who teach in undergraduate nursing programs have tended to rely on the written nursing care plan or its variants as a way to teach and evaluate the skills of clinical judgment. Presumably the written care plan reflects the thinking processes which the student has used in deciding on nursing action and represents the application of theoretical knowledge to practice. Yet most of us would agree that the care plan lacks efficiency as an instructional method and there is no empirical evidence as to its effectiveness.

Educational methodologists have long argued that the development of strategies to teach any task rests on an analysis of how competent individuals perform that task (Taba and Elzey, 1964; Glaser, 1976). Hence, an understanding of the cognitive processes employed by expert clinicians in making a judgment may assist us in developing more precise and efficient instructional strategies to teach these processes to individual learners. The linear sequence of thought defined by the nursing process may not, in fact, capture the thought processes actually employed to make sound clinical judgments. Analysis of those thought processes should put us in a better position to teach them.

The primary objectives of this chapter are: 1) to review and evaluate the research literature which describes the cognitive processes of clinical judgment and 2) to derive from the literature suggestions for educators attempting to help their students become astute clinical judges. Research on measurement of clinical judgment skills is not included, except as it pertains to the descriptive studies. The reader interested in assessment of judgment skill is referred to the review by Tanner (1978) and the recent investigations reported by Holzemer and associates (1981) and McLaughlin and associates (1979, 1980, 1981).

Two important points should be kept in mind while reading this review. First, the research on clinical judgment is largely descriptive. A portrayal of how competent individuals make clinical judgments does not automatically translate to a definition of the thinking processes we should teach our students nor by what methods we should teach them. Further research would be necessary to translate the descriptive theory to prescriptions for teaching. Secondly, the majority of the clinical judgment research focuses on medical judgment, using physicians and medical students as subjects. There are a few studies on nurses, and most of these use tasks which fall within the medical domain. It is widely assumed that while the *content* of the judgment may differ, the *process* of judgment is the same, regardless of discipline orientation. This assumption is derived from: 1) the similarity in the uncertain, high-risk, probabilistic nature of any clinical judgment task and 2) theoretical support for invariant characteristics of human judges, regardless of the task.

Review of Literature on Clinical Judgment
Overview

Research on the processes of clinical judgment may be classified along three dimensions: 1) by the component of the judgment process studied, 2) by the variables examined which influence both the judgment process and its outcome and 3) by the theoretical perspective and related research methods used as the basis for the study.

The process of clinical judgment is typically viewed as a series of decisions including: 1) decisions regarding *what* to observe in the patient situation, 2) inferential decisions, deriving meaning from data observed (diagnosis) and 3) decisions regarding actions which should be taken that will be of optimal benefit to the patient (management). Research on clinical judgment tends to focus on one of these three components, with the vast majority of investigations centering on the inferential reasoning of diagnosis and the interaction between observation or data gathering strategies and diagnosis.

The second dimension for classifying clinical judgment research is composed of the variables which influence both the process and the outcome of clinical judgments:

1) *Task variables* define the overall complexity of the situation including the amount and nature of the information available to the clinician, the number of problems the patient may be experiencing, the courses of action available.

2) *Contextual variables* include the circumstances and setting in which the clinical judgment is made; these are factors which may not be immediately apparent in the presenting situation but may nevertheless influence both the judgment process and its outcome. This category includes variables such as institutional policy, characteristics of the patient's physician, and time available to make the judgment.

3) *Clinician variables* represent the host of characteristics the decision-maker brings to the task, such as attitudes and values, past experience with similar tasks, clinical knowledge and level of inferential ability.

4) *Risk/benefit variables* are those associated with the judgment itself, including both the risks and potential benefits associated with any action chosen by the clinician. For example, in medical judgments, a physician attempting to diagnose the cause of hypertension must weigh the risk and potential benefits to the patient before recommending an arteriogram. A nurse, in helping a family make decisions about institutionalization of an elderly family member, must consider the probable consequences of such action.

Most research on clinical judgment uses simulated tasks (i.e. patient situations represented by written or filmed case studies). Although efforts are made to simulate real-life clinical encounters, the use of simulations limits the capacity to examine the influence of either the contextual variables or the risk-benefit variables. In some studies there has been effort to either control or at least describe task variables, but in only one study has task complexity been varied systematically. The most comprehensive investigations of clinician variables have included comparisons of judgment processes between novices and experts. There have been isolated studies of personality characteristics and measures of inferential ability as

3

they relate to clinical judgment.

The third dimension for classifying research on clinical judgment is the theoretical perspective and its associated research paradigm. The majority of clinical judgment research has generated from either decision theory or information processing theory. Although the two approaches purportedly investigate the processes of clinical judgment, they vary greatly in the extent to which they strive to make public the actual intellectual processes which would otherwise be unobservable. As would be expected, they also vary in the research methods employed and in the components of the process and associated variables which are examined.

Students of clinical judgment as a decision-making process rely heavily on mathematical or statistical models to: 1) make explicit the decision-maker's policies in weighing various cues to make a diagnosis or in assigning values and probabilities to outcomes in management decisions or 2) use as a comparison to the judge's actual performance. Students of clinical judgment within the information-processing paradigm place more emphasis on describing and/or explaining the actual processes employed rather than attempting to represent them mathematically. Consistency with other components of information processing theory, most notably current notions of memory structure and processes, is an integral part of this view of clinical judgment.

The following review of literature uses the two theoretical perspectives as a means of organizing the research completed. For each, there is further exploration of underlying theory, a description and critique of methods employed and a description of individual studies emphasizing the component of the process and the categories of variables examined. Educational implications which are suggested by investigators and studies of instructional strategies derived from each theoretical perspective are also reviewed and evaluated.

Decision - Theory

Decision - theory seeks to describe or prescribe how individuals or groups choose a course of action. The choice is made under conditions of varying degrees of certainty about the probable outcomes of actions and varying degrees of risk associated with the action (Albert, 1978). Applications of decision-theory to clinical judgment have been primarily prescriptive decision analysis — how an individual *should* make a decision. The probabilistic nature of clinical decision making lends itself to statistical modeling approaches. The normative or prescriptive theory attempts to describe mathematically how judges should: 1) weight cues to derive a diagnosis or 2) choose an action which has the highest probability of achieving the most highly valued outcome.

In the typical experiment in decision analysis, the subject is presented with a simulated case study. He is asked to assign "subjective probabilities" to elements within the case. In studies of diagnosis, the subject is asked to assign probabilities to tentative diagnoses and to cues in relation to each diagnosis. In studies on selection of management strategies, the subject is asked to assign probabilities of the occurrence of certain outcomes given certain actions and to estimate the value or risk of each outcome. Mathematical models using the subjectively assigned values prescribe what the judgment, either diagnosis or management, should be. The theory is tested by a comparison of the judgment actually made by the clinician and that derived by the mathematical model. Three general approaches have been employed in mathematical modeling of clinical decisions: Brunswik's lens model, Bayes Theorem, and Utility Theory.

THE LENS MODEL   The lens model represents probabilistic interrelations between human and environmental components of the judgment situation. Figure 1 depicts the lens model applied by Hammond (1964, p. 317) to the study of clinical inference in nursing. There is a state of the patient (SP) which is unknown and can only be inferred by the cues (signs and symptoms) the patient displays. The relationships between the cues and the SP are uncertain and probabilistic, e.g. the presence of some cue probably indicates the presence of some condition while the absence of the cue may or may not indicate the absence of the condition. Presumably the nurse has some knowledge about possible SP's and some knowledge about the relationship between cues and the SP. The left portion of the box represents the "signal receiving" system of the nurse — the past experience, knowledge, etc. which may influence the nurse's attention to the value assigned to cues.

Figure 1
Application of Lens Model
to Clinical Influence
(Hammond, 1964, p. 317)

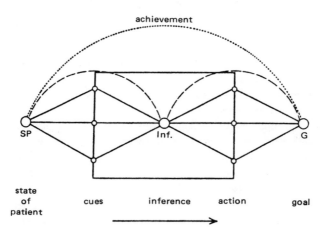

The right side of the diagram is the action-system of the nurse. As there are many cues suggestive of any given SP, there are multiple actions which may achieve a single goal. Once again there is an uncertain, probabilistic relationship between the actions and the desired goal. The "lens" is the past experience, knowledge, etc. of the clinician through which cues and possible actions are filtered.

The lens model was used by Hammond (1966) in a thoughtful analysis of the complexity of diagnostic tasks — tasks in which the nurse must "... infer correctly the impalpable state of the patient from the uncertain, palpable data presented by the patient" (p. 29). The most simple of diagnostics tasks is that in which a state of the patient can be ascertained as present or absent by the presence or absence of a single cue; in such a case, the cue has a certain, high probability relationship to the diagnosis. The most difficult task is differential diagnoses in which there are multiple possible states of the patient and multiple cues, each with a probabilistic relationship to the state of patient. A number of other characteristics of multiple cues, uncertainty-geared inference tasks also contribute to task complexity.

In a now classic series of studies, Hammond and associates attempted to apply the lens model and this task analysis to the study of: 1) the cognitive tasks representative of nursing problems (1966a), 2) the information units used in making a diagnostic inference (1966b), and 3) the information seeking strategies used for diagnostic inference (1966c).

The first field study attempted to define the cognitive tasks, their frequency and the cue characteristics of the more frequently occurring tasks (Hammond et al, 1966a). Forty-seven hospital nurses were asked to record for a 24-hour period situations which required a clinical inference and decision. The result was a large number of varied decision situations which could not be analyzed in terms of cue clusters. A second field study reported in the same publication (Hammond et al, 1966a) focused on a single situation — complaint of abdominal pain following abdominal surgery — tabulating frequency of occurrence in the 30 surveyed hospitals and analyzing actions taken by nurses in response to patient's complaint. Fifteen action categories were identified in 212 cases. There was no significant relationship between any one cue and selection of any of the action categories; this was interpreted to mean that no single cue transmitted a significant amount of information with respect to the action category selected.

To further analyze the information used by a nurse to make an inferential judgment, Hammond and associates conducted an intensive study of six nurses (Hammond et al, 1966b). The major purpose of the study was to identify what basic units of information (i.e. single cues to categories of cues) were associated with selection of certain action categories. The six nurses responded to 100 cases selected from those developed in the second field study (Hammond et al 1966a). Cues were treated singly or grouped as cue configurations based on textbook descriptions and on categories selected by the nurse as useful. Subjects were also asked to identify the degree of confidence in their inferences. As in the previous study, no single cue was found to be related to the selection of action, nor were any groupings related to the inferences made. It was also found that the nurse subjects did not consciously discriminate among the usefulness of various cues. Their confidence in their inferences varied little over the cases. It is interesting to note that even though basic message units are taught (nurses presumably learn clusters of cues associated with certain states of patients), these units were evidently not employed by nurses to decide on a course of action.

Despite methodological flaws cited by the investigators, this series of studies, as the only explicit effort to analyze the structural characteristics of the task, has made an important contribution to the study of clinical judgment. The recognition of the complexity of the judgment process, the identification of variation among subjects and the provision of a beginning framework for analyzing task complexity are significant contributions.

BAYES THEOREM   Bayes theorem is a statistical model which describes the way in which judgments are revised in light of new information. It originated with Reverend Thomas Bayes in 1763 and interest in it was revived by Savage in 1954.

Savage fused the concepts of utility and personal probability into a theory of decision in the face of uncertainty, "a highly idealized theory of the behavior of a 'rational' person with respect to decisions" (Savage, 1954, p.7).

Bayes' theorem was first introduced to the study of medical judgment by Ledley and Lusted (1959) who described the parallels between its logic and the informal processes of diagnostic reasoning. A clinician entertains a diagnostic hypothesis about the state of the patient given a cue. For example, the nurse may have identified elevated temperature in the postoperative patient and entertained the hypothesis of infection. S/he would assign a probability to the hypothesis 'infection' given the cue 'temperature elevation'.

The revision of the likelihood of diagnostic hypothesis given the cue is based on three additional statements:

1. The prior probability of the hypothesis without reference to a cue, or the unconditional probability. In the example above, the incidence (or its estimate) of postoperative infection would constitute this probability denoted $p(H)$.

2. The probability of a cue (sign or symptom) given a certain diagnostic hypothesis $p(C/H)$. In this case, it would be the estimate of incidence of fever in patients with postoperative infection.

3. The probability of a cue without reference to a diagnostic hypothesis $p(C)$. In this case, $p(C)$ would be an estimate of the incidence of fever regardless of diagnostic possibilities — or stated another way the incidence of fever in the sum of all possible diagnoses:

$$p(H/C) = \Sigma \ i \ (^H i) \ p(^C i/^H i)$$

Bayes' theorem describes the process of revising the probability of a diagnostic hypothesis given a cue $p(H/C)$ by combining the prior probabilities of a diagnosis $p(H)$, and of a single cue, $p(C)$, and the conditional probability of a cue's occurrence given the diagnostic hypothesis $p(C/H)$:

$$p(H/C) = p(H) \ p(C)$$

The posterior probability $p(H/C)$ is subject to revision as the clinician accumulates data. According to Kozielecki (1972) in his efforts to apply the Bayesian model to diagnosis, it is the revision of posterior probabilities that constitutes a major part of the diagnostic process. In Kozielecki's model, when the most probable hypothesis reaches some diagnostic threshold it is accepted as the diagnosis.

The application of Bayes model to clinical judgment is not an attempt to model identically the judgment process. Rather it seeks to determine the extent to which "intuitive" clinical judgments match the optimal process described by Bayes model. It is unlikely that human judges do the mental gymnastics espoused in Bayes model, but that in all likelihood some informal probability assignment is used both in inferential judgments like diagnosis and in judgments about alternative courses of action.

Two early studies attempted to apply the Bayesian model to the study of the diagnostic process. Hammond and his associates (1967) examined the self-consistency in probability revision and the accuracy of the revision as dictated by Bayes model. Six nurses were given 12 cases judged typical of nursing inferential

7

tasks. Each case was a binomial diagnostic task; i.e. the nurses had to judge whether a given condition was present or absent. The subjects were given a brief patient description and a possible patient condition. They were asked to state the prior probability of the condition, select data one cue at a time, state conditional probability, then given the data, state the revision of the probability of the condition in light of the new data. The subjective probability estimates were used in Bayes model and the subjects' performance in probability revision was compared with the product of the model. The results were strikingly similar to the majority of laboratory studies on probability revision; the nurses tended to revise probabilities in the direction dictated by Bayes' theorem but the amount of revision was much less than that prescribed. In addition, the nurse subjects tended to revise probabilities in a self-consistent manner.

Kozielecki (1970) attempted to design an experiment representative of a medical diagnostic task yet retaining laboratory-type experimental control. In this experiment, subjects were required to identify one of 21 alternative diseases in a patient. Each was defined as the combination of two symptoms from among seven possible symptoms: A,B,C,D,E,F, and G. Thus, the diseases were AB, AC, AD, etc. All diseases were of the same prior probability. While working on the diagnosis, the subjects performed medical tests which supplied them with probabilistic information on the symptoms. The conditional probability was equal to either 0.70 or 0.30. Throughout the diagnosing, the subjects were given 10 successive data or symptoms.

After each new datum, the subjects revised probability estimates of each of a small number of hypotheses, "modal hypotheses," and the total of the remaining hypotheses, "the catchall". For example, a subject may assign the following probabilities to three hypotheses from the system of modal hypotheses: p(AB) = 0.40, p(CD) = 0.20, p(DF) = 0.20; then, the probability of the remaining 18 hypotheses in the catchall was 0.20.

The result of this experiment suggested a tendency toward overestimation of conditional probabilities, termed "radicalism" by Kozielecki. He suggested that radicalism is a function of the size of the hypothesis pool — with wide inference tasks, one tends to overestimate conditional probabilities, while with narrow tasks (few hypotheses) the tendency is toward conservatism.

In an effort to further analyze the common phenomenon of conservatism in revising probabilities, Tversky and Kahneman (1973, 1974, Kahneman and Tversky, 1972) conducted several studies examining methods of assigning subjective probabilities. While the judgment tasks were not clinical in nature, they required use of information the subject brought to the experiment — his own knowledge — and therefore there may be some corollary to clinical inference tasks.

In Bayesian paradigm-type studies, Tversky and Kahneman reported evidence of the use of two heuristics governing assignment of subjective probabilities: availability and representativeness. Availability of instances refers to the strategy by which people assess the frequency of a class or the probability of an event by the ease with which it is brought to mind. For example, one may assess the risk of heart attack among middle-aged people by recalling such occurrences among one's acquaintances. Availability clearly has utility as a heuristic for assessing frequency or probability because instances of high frequency classes are usually recalled better and more quickly than those of low frequency classes. However, availability can be biased by a number of other factors besides frequency or probability.

One such bias, retrievability of instances, seems particularly applicable to diagnosis. In an experiment demonstrating this (Tversky and Kahneman, 1973), subjects were read a list of well-known personalities of both sexes and were subsequently asked to judge whether the list contained more names of men than women. Different lists were used, some of which contained names of men who were more famous than the women, and others in which the names of the women were more famous than the men. In each case the subjects erroneously judged the more numerous class to be that which held the more famous personalities.

It is plausible that similar biases may be introduced by the use of this heuristic in diagnosis. Recent encounters with patients suffering from a specific disorder may increase the subjective probability of that disease in subsequent encounters. Similarly, the impact of a particular patient's death or prolonged disability may increase the subjective probability of the underlying disorder. Shiffman and her associates (1978) conducted a study to assess the extent to which availability is used as a heuristic in selecting initial diagnostic hypotheses. Eight brief cases were presented to a sample of 34 internists. Subjects were asked to generate tentative diagnoses, listing them in the order in which they were recalled, (defined as availability) to estimate probabilities of each of the tentative diagnoses and to rate the seriousness of each diagnosis. It was found that the availability order of tentative diagnoses was highly related to the physician's probability estimate but not to their ratings of seriousness. The physician's probability estimate in turn, was not uniformly correlated with probabilities based on actuarial data. The investigators concluded that availability is used as a heuristic in diagnostic tasks and that its use may distort the physician's diagnostic judgments.

The second heuristic reported by Tversky and Kahneman (1974) is that of representativeness. According to this heuristic, the subjective probability of an event, or a sample, is determined by "the degree to which it: 1) is similar in essential characteristics to the parent population, and 2) reflects the salient features of the process by which it is generated"(p. 430.)

Tversky and Kahneman (1974) demonstrated that people generally ignore the prior probabilities of outcomes when given other data. Subjects were shown personality descriptions of several individuals, allegedly drawn at random from a group of 100 professionals — engineers and lawyers. The subjects were asked to estimate the probability, for each description, that it belonged to an engineer rather than a lawyer. In one experimental condition, the subjects were told that the group from which the description had been drawn was comprised of 70 engineers and 30 lawyers. In another condition, they were told that the sample consisted of 30 engineers and 70 lawyers. The subjects in the two groups produced essentially the same probability judgments, in complete violation of Bayes' rule. This was interpreted to mean that the subjects evaluated the probabilities by the degree to which the description was representative of one of the two stereotypes, virtually ignoring the prior probabilities.

Although there is no empirical evidence, it seems likely on logical grounds that a similar heuristic may be employed in medical diagnosis. If a set of cues is deemed representative of one disorder more than another, any knowledge of prior probabilities may be ignored.

Following their research on representativeness, Tversky and Kahneman summarized the relationship of their findings to the Bayesian model:

> The usefulness of the normative Bayesian approach to the analysis and the modeling of subjective probability lies not on the accuracy of the subjective estimates, but rather on whether the model captures the essential determinates of the judgment process. The research discussed in this paper suggests that it does not... In his evaluation of evidence, man is apparently not a conservative Bayesian: he is not a Bayesian at all. (Kahneman and Tversky, 1972, p. 353).

UTILITY THEORY   Utility theory describes the selection of an action or set of actions based on a subjective assignment of value to probable outcomes of those actions. It is designed to optimize decision making under conditions of risk — prescribing the choice that maximizes expected utility or value. When a clinician is faced with a decision problem, there are a set of actions (management strategies) from which s/he may select. Each action is associated with a set of possible outcomes and each outcome, in turn, is associated with both a probability of occurrence (p) and a value assignment or utility function (V). The expected value for each *outcome* is the probability multiplied by the value. The expected value (EV) for each *action* is the sum of all expected values for all the possible outcomes of the action:

$$EV = \Sigma \ i \ (P \ X \ V) \qquad i = outcomes$$

The optimal decision produced by the model is the action with the highest expected value.

As in Bayesian studies, utility model is tested by a comparison of the judge's actual decision with that derived from the model. Unlike the application of the Bayesian model to diagnosis, this model produces a single expected value, rather than changing probabilities. And unlike the Bayesian applications, utility theory allows for inclusion of both contextual variables in the subjective probability assignments and risk/benefit variables in the subjective assignment of value.

Grier (1976) is the only investigator who has extended utility theory to the study of clinical judgment in nursing. The purpose of her study was to determine if intuitive decisions by nurses were in agreement with those prescribed by the model. The 50 nurse subjects were presented with four patient situations. They were asked first to rank order from best to poorest three possible courses of action (the intuitive judgment). They were then asked to estimate the probability that each of seven outcomes would occur given each of three actions (a total of 21 probabilities). They also were asked to assign a value for each of the outcomes, numerically rated and totalling 100 points for all outcomes. A total of 185 decisions were analyzed. Nurses' intuitive judgments agreed with the quantitatively derived preferred action in 109 (58.9%) of the cases. The agreement was statistically significant on three of the four cases. The correlation between the rank orderings of intuitively derived actions and those of quantitatively derived actions were all statistically significant but ranged from a Tau of .25 to .82. Grier concluded that these findings provide evidence that "decision theory is applicable to nursing" (p. 109). She further suggested that a "...systematic and objective process was used in making most of the decisions, resulting in a justifiable choice of action for achieving the desired goal" (p. 108). What in unaccounted for in these findings is the process used to derive the remaining 41% of the decisions.

EDUCATIONAL IMPLICATIONS OF DECISION-THEORY   Many investigators would agree that neither the Bayesian model nor utility theory are accurate representations of the actual judgment process (e.g. Slovic and Lichtenstein, 1971; Kahneman and Tversky, 1972; Albert, 1978). Several investigators have suggested that the accuracy of diagnosis may be improved by use of Bayesian model, especially when actuarial data can be used in combination subjective probability estimation. Schwartz et al (1973) advocated instruction in quantitative aspects of decision-theory and statistical modeling. They further suggested that clinical judgments (both diagnostic and management) could be improved by the construction and use of decision trees which display the diagnostic probabilities as well as risks and expected values associated with diagnostic procedures and medical and surgical interventions. They acknowledge the obvious difficulty in constructing decision trees for the large domain of medical decision-making. Although the ability to quantitatively formalize medical decisions may ultimately improve practice, the notion of decision-tree construction and their use has not come to fruition.

In the one study in nursing attempting to translate decision theory into instructional strategy, Aspinall (1979) tested the effectiveness of using decision trees to improve nurses' diagnostic accuracy. Thirty triads of nurses, matched for educational background, length of experience and previous performance comprised one experimental and two control groups. All subjects were given a written case study and were asked to list all possible diagnoses which could cause the change in behavior exhibited by the patient. Experimental group nurses were given a set of binary decision trees to enable them to use information systematically and to determine if characteristics of each condition were present. Significant improvement in ability to identify possible diagnoses was shown by nurses who used the decision trees.

Presumably the use of a decision tree might be instructive to students in formal aspects of clinical inference. From their use, students may then learn the process of clinical inference which would assist them in the majority of tasks where decision trees are not available. Aspinall's study did not examine the extent to which the experimental nurses' performance was improved under conditions where decision trees were unavailable.

Grier (1976) draws educational implications from her study of clinical decision-making. She suggests that nurses should be taught a procedure for making decisions "... because decision theory focuses on essential aspects of the nursing process" (p. 109). She further suggests that nurses should be encouraged to use the model of clinical decision making employed in her study, implying that the result will be improved patient care.

These inferences have at least two serious flaws. First in Grier's study there was no effort to determine whether or not the chosen action, either the intuitively or the quantitatively derived action, would in fact result in a desired outcome. Nursing, unlike much of medicine, lacks sufficient scientific base to predictably link outcomes to actions. The results of Grier's study were based on subjectively assigned estimates and indicate only that in the slight majority of decisions nurses' intuitive decisions matched the quantitative decisions, not that they were better decisions in terms of actual patient outcomes. Secondly, the tasks were constructed with a limited range of outcomes and limited set of actions, hence a *closed* task. This is rarely the case in actual practice where the range of outcomes and actions is almost unlimited.

The studies of Grier, Aspinall, Hammond and associates, and Kozielecki all indicate that the performance of the clinical decision-maker does not match that prescribed by the statistical model. The work of Kahneman and Tversky and Schiffman et al. provide some explanation of the discrepancy between human and statistical decision-making in terms of biases introduced by the human. Two educational approaches may be useful in improving clinical judgment and warrant investigation. One is to introduce formal decision-theory methods as attempted by Aspinall or as suggested by Grier to assist students to become more systematic in consideration of alternatives. A second approach is to help students recognize biases which they may bring to the decision situation so that the untoward influence of such biases can be reduced or their utility optimized. The latter approach is one which is also supported by studies in the information processing paradigm as we shall see in the following discussion.

Information Processing Theory

Information-processing theory has its roots in the work of Simon and Newell in artificial intelligence (Newell, Shaw and Simon, 1958; Simon, 1978; Newell and Simon, 1972). An extensive theory of human problem-solving has evolved from use of verbal protocol analysis and subsequent computer programming.

The theory describes problem-solving behavior as an interaction between an information-processing system (the problem-solver) and a task environment (the task as described by the experimenter). The major assumption underlying the theory is that there are limits to human information processing capacity; effective problem-solving rests on the system's ability to *adapt* to these limitations. Two types of limitations are critical: factors which determine the amount of information to which the human can attend at one time and factors which determine the clarity and accessibility of the information either in the task environment or internal to the problem-solver (e.g. failure to remember the meaning of important clinical data). With most tasks, performance is limited by internal factors, primarily in the amount of information one can attend to.

This limitation is derived from the small capacity of the working memory (commonly referred to as the short-term memory or STM). Miller (1956), in a now classic series of studies, found that the STM holds an invariant number of symbols (7 $\pm$ 2). The capacity of the STM can be dramatically increased by coding familiar stimulus patterns into simple units: for example, the sequence P-E-N is coded as a single unit while E-P-N is coded as three separate units.

In complex tasks, with large amounts of information, such as diagnosis, the resource requirements are tremendous and the problem-solver may experience "cognitive strain" (Bruner et al, 1956). Such strain can be reduced by use of heuristics — shortcut strategies to achieve problem-resolution. For example, the cognitive strain imposed by large amounts of clinical data may be reduced by clustering the data into diagnostic hypotheses. The heuristics described by Schiffman and associates (1981) in assessing probability of diagnoses are another example of mechanisms to reduce cognitive strain. In addition, specific cognitive strategies may be used in familiar or recurring tasks in order to reduce the information processing demands.

Clinical judgment research based on information processing theory has attempted to describe how clinicians adapt to the demands of a complex task environment. The focus of virtually all investigations within this paradigm has been on the cognitive strategies employed by expert and novice clinicians in deriving a diagnosis.

The experimental methods used within this framework are derivatives of Newell and Simon's verbal protocol analysis. The subject is presented with a simulation, of varying degrees of fidelity to an actual patient situation. In some studies, the simulation is in the form of an actor trained to provide a history and to present signs and symptoms representative of a real patient. In others, it is presented as a brief videotaped vignette, portraying the initial part of the clinician-patient encounter, while yet in others, it is a written case study. The use of simulated patients rather than actual patients permits control over the cues presented as well as comparison of a performance across subjects.

Subjects are instructed to proceed in a diagnostic work-up with the trained actor as they would with a real patient; for videotaped or written case studies, subjects ask for information, one cue at a time, from an examiner, as if they were eliciting the information from the patient. Both concurrent and retrospective verbal protocols are employed. In concurrent, subjects are instructed to "think-aloud" as they proceed through the work-up, explaining their rationale behind questioning as they proceed. In retrospective verbal protocols, a "stimulated recall" method is generally employed in which subjects listen to a tape recording (or observe a videotape) of the work-up and describe what their thinking was with each cue elicited. Both the diagnostic work-up approach and the verbal protocols are tape-recorded, transcribed and generally used in both quantitative and descriptive analysis. In some studies, the verbal protocols have been translated into computer programs as a means to describe and/or test diagnostic reasoning strategies (Kleinmuntz, 1963, 1968; Wortman, 1972).

This method of investigation was first introduced to the study of diagnostic reasoning by Kleinmuntz (1963) and employed in an extensive series of studies reported by Elstein and associates (1972, 1978). A general model of diagnostic problem-solving has evolved and is the one which is the major focus of most studies within the information processing framework. Occupying a central position within this model is the notion of generation of diagnostic hypotheses very early in the work-up (Elstein, et al, 1972). According to the model, the clinician attends to initially available relevant cues. From these few cues, diagnostic possibilities are activated at a level specifically appropriate to the cues. Subsequent data gathering is generally hypothesis directed; that is, additional data is gathered with the goal of ruling in, ruling out or furthering refining hypotheses. Each hypothesis is continually evaluated in light of each new cue.

The tenet of early hypothesis activation in this model is an important one both from a theoretical and a practical perspective. The use of the so-called hypothetico-deductive approach to diagnosis is explained, in terms of information processing theory, as the primary way that the clinician adapts his limited resources to the demands of the task environment. It is argued that early hypotheses serve as a "chunking" mechanism in short-term memory, greatly increasing its capacity to hold the huge amounts of clinical data acquired in the diagnostic work-up (Elstein, 1978). Hence, it is reasoned, that it is likely that all clinicians use this as a primary strategy in diagnosis because it assists in conserving the limited information processing resources.

In addition to its consistency with general information processing theory, the notion of early hypothesis generation also represents a point of convergence with decision-theory. Bayesian theory assumes the presence of hypotheses, the probability of which are revised during the diagnostic work-up.

From the practical standpoint, traditional instruction in clinical problem solving is diametrically opposed to the use of early diagnostic hypotheses. Students are typically instructed to systematically collect all data, withholding any judgment, then to proceed in an unprejudiced analysis of the data to a logical conclusion. If early hypothesis generation is a common strategy employed by clinicians, then more effective instruction might be developed which would assist students to optimally use this strategy.

Despite the apparent theoretical support for the general model of diagnostic problem-solving, the methods used to derive it have some serious shortcomings which must be considered in evaluating the literature. First, the protocol analysis relies on verbal reports of subjects and it is not known whether higher-level mental processes are truly accessible to the subject (Nisbett and Wilson, 1977). Proponents of the method argue that verbal reports of thinking do provide indirect evidence of the underlying processes which produce them. However, the extent to which the very process of thinking aloud alters the content and process of thought is not known (Neisser, 1968). Ericsson and Simon (1980) introduced evidence that verbalizing information affects cognitive processes only if the instructions require verbalization of information that would not otherwise be attended to; this may well be the case in studies of clinical judgment, and the problem may be only partially remedied by retrospective verbal protocols.

The second shortcoming is that verbal protocols produce huge amounts of data. The method is generally used with a small number of simulations and a small number of subjects. Efforts to find either task specific patterns of judgment processes across subjects or generic strategies which occur across tasks are severely constrained.

The third limitation is related to validity and is a problem inherent in the use of simulation. It is not possible to portray in a simulation all the cues to which a subject responds. Dreyfus (1979) points out that many of these cues are on the "fringes of consciousness" in terms of their use in problem solving. Their importance to the task may be unrecognized by both those constructing the simulation and the subjects responding to the simulation. Similarly, contextual as well as risk/benefit variables, which may profoundly influence the judgment process, are typically not considered. In sum, the extent to which the judgment process portrayed in verbal protocols is a valid representation of process used in actual practice is not known.

Studies using the verbal protocol method and based on information processing theory have been conducted to: (1) test the general model of diagnostic reasoning with experts and novices, (2) further describe the thinking strategies used by clinicians in information seeking hypothesis activation, (3) describe the relationship of the task environment to the strategies employed, (4) identify correlates of diagnostic skill, and (5) test teaching methods designed to improve use of selected cognitive strategies.

GENERAL MODEL OF DIAGNOSTIC REASONING   The most extensive series of studies to develop and test a general model of diagnostic reasoning was conducted by Elstein and associates (1972, 1978). The studies were designed specifically to: (1) determine how medical diagnostic problems are solved, (2) identify processes which characterize the thinking of expert physicians as contrasted with nonexperts, (3) define the processes which distinguish accurate from inaccurate diagnostic outcomes, (4) determine how early diagnostic hypotheses are generated and how extensive a data base is needed, (5) identify the decision rules used to confirm or eliminate hypotheses, and (6) describe the most common errors in diagnostic reasoning (Elstein, et al, 1978, pp. 66-67).

The initial study used trained actors for three simulated diagnostic work-ups with periodic concurrent thinking aloud as well as stimulated recall methods. The sample was comprised of a total of 24 physicians, 17 of whom were "criterial" (i.e. nominated by at least five peers as expert diagnosticians) and seven of whom were "non-criterial" physicians (i.e. nominated by fewer than five peers). The processes employed for each case were described, errors of diagnosis were analyzed, and scores were obtained on twelve dependent variables. Findings of this study can be summarized as follows:

1. Hypothesis generation begins about ten percent of the way through a work-up.
2. Some medical problems are approached by generating specific hypothesis early, others by a progression from general to specific — a feature which appears to be more task dependent than related to individual problem-solving style.
3. The total number of hypotheses considered varied from 4 to 7, a finding interpreted as supporting the notion that hypotheses serve as a chunking mechanism, conserving limited space in STM.
4. There were no significant differences between critical and non-critical physicians on the point of generation of hypotheses, total number of hypotheses generated, percentage of cues acquired, efficiency or accuracy of cue interpretation. These findings may be accounted for by the process of selection of criterial and noncriterial physicians.
5. Diagnostic accuracy was found to be associated with thoroughness in cue acquisition and accuracy of cue interpretation.
6. There was no consistency across or within the three tasks, or across or within the physicians in processes or rules used to determine acceptance of a diagnostic hypothesis.

In summary, the only general strategies which were consistent across physicians and tasks were early hypothesis generation and data gathering to test diagnostic hypotheses.

In a second study, Elstein and associates (1978) continued their search for a set of diagnostic strategies which were common across tasks and diagnosticians. Fifteen of the 24 physicians in the original study completed four paper-and-pencil simulations called patient-management problems (PMPs). The PMP begins with a brief description of the patient's problem. The examiner must then decide what, if any, work-up is indicated. If he chooses further work-up, he is presented with a long list of questions that yield information about a patient. The examinee selects questions (e.g history, physical exam data) by erasing an opaque overlay on a specially constructed answer sheet, revealing the data requested. On the bases of these data, decisions are made on the next steps to be taken.

As in the first study by Elstein and associates (1972, 1978), there was evidence that hypothesis generation occurred very early and that the hypotheses influenced the data selected. However, rates of data acquisition and hypothesis generation varied considerably with each problem. There was also considerable within-individual variation, suggesting that physicians do not apply self-consistent strategies, but that the strategy itself varies depending on the problem.

What Elstein and associates have termed the "ubiquitous phenomenon of early hypotheses-generation" has been corroborated in studies of physicians by Barrows and Bennett (1972), and Kassirer and Gorry (1978), in studies of medical students by Neufeld et al (1981), Ekwo et al (1977), and to a lesser extent in a study of nursing students by Tanner (1977). Each of these studies will be briefly reviewed.

Barrows and Bennett (1972) studied the thinking processes of six neurologists. They used simulated patient encounters and analyzed the written work-up, as well as videotapes of the encounter using a stimulated recall method. They reported the "appearance of hypotheses in the neurologist's mind almost before the interview begins" based on patient appearance, age, sex, dress, manner and the patient's response to one or two questions (p. 275).

Kassirer and Gorry (1978) studied six clinicians - four nephrologists, a cardiologist and a gastroenterologist using a simulated patient and concurrent thinking aloud during the diagnostic work-up. Like Elstein and associates, Barrows and Bennett found that subjects generated hypotheses very early in the history taking process. While the total number of hypotheses ranged from 14 to 37, the subjects indicated that they maintained 4 to 11 hypotheses active at any one time. Kassirer and Gorry also report that the process of hypothesis activation dominated the early part of the encounter, while later in the session the emphasis was on hypothesis evaluation.

Also using a simulated patient and both concurrent thinking aloud and stimulated recall methods, Ekwo (1977) studied the diagnostic reasoning of 20 junior medical students. Students were tested on two problems — one of familiar clinical content, the other of "non-familiar" content. Early hypothesis generation occurred with both problems, but more often in the familiar problem.

In a longitudinal and cross-sectional study, Neufeld and associates (1981) examined the development of clinical problem-solving skills in medical students. A cross-sectional sample of 35 students selected from three classes were examined; in addition 22 students were observed at four yearly intervals to the first postgraduate year. The students conducted a diagnostic work-up of four simulated patients; "stimulated recall" methods were used as in other studies. It was found that early hypothesis generation was characteristic of students at all educational levels, and that the initial hypothesis is generated by all student samples on the average within 30 seconds of eliciting the chief complaint. There was a small difference in average specificity of hypotheses with the younger students using more general hypotheses. The hypothesis aggregate score, a measure of the similarity between the subject's hypothesis and a pool of ideal hypotheses, was significantly related to educational level.

Tanner (1977) in a study of instructional methods examined the diagnostic strategies of 54 senior baccalaureate nursing students. The subjects responded to five short videotaped vignettes of hospitalized patients; subjects were instructed to think aloud as they sought information from the examiner and proceeded in their problem-solving. Subjects generated from one to six hypotheses immediately after viewing the videotape. Although this finding may have been an artifact of the testing situation, there was also evidence that subjects were using hypotheses to direct their subsequent information-seeking. A small positive relationship was found between diagnostic accuracy and the number of early diagnostic hypotheses. However, the major determinant of diagnostic accuracy was whether or not the correct diagnosis was included in the initial set of hypotheses.

In summary, the only consistent diagnostic strategy which has been found to occur across subjects and tasks is early hypothesis generation and testing. Only one study examined this strategy in nursing students and it is not known whether the use of the strategy by nursing students would persist under differing testing conditions.

INFORMATION-SEEKING STRATEGIES Six studies have examined the information-seeking strategies used in diagnostic reasoning. All but one have assumed generally that a hypothesis testing strategy of some kind is employed, and the resulting descriptions are couched within that context.

In both the high-fidelity situations and the PMPs, Elstein and associates (1978) attempted to find data acquisition strategies which were consistent across tasks or within subjects. They found no consistency in variables of cue acquisition, critical findings or efficiency of data gathering. Thoroughness in cue acquisition and accuracy of cue interpretation were associated with diagnostic accuracy and hence are important components of information gathering.

Kassirer and Gorry (1978), in their study of six physicians, described the process of "case building" as being comprised of four general strategies used to seek information and evaluate remaining hypotheses. Like Elstein and associates, they assumed that data gathering was generally conducted through hypothesis testing, so the description of strategies is couched in that context. Among these strategies are: (a) a confirmation strategy in which the clinician seeks data which would prove a hypothesis, by matching the characteristics of the clinical state under consideration, (b) an *elimination* strategy that uses questions about findings which are so often found with a given disease that their absence weighs heavily against the hypothesized disease, (c) a discrimination strategy used to distinguish one hypothesis from another, and (d) an exploration strategy used to refine a hypothesis by making it more specific and by checking for related or unrelated disorders or complications.

Barrows and Bennett (1972) in their study of neurologists described two general types of questioning approaches — "inquiry-oriented", hypothesis testing questions and questions that are part of a routine inquiry. They suggest that inquiry-oriented questions begin as soon as hypotheses are activated but that physicians switch to routine questioning in one of three conditions: (1) when the inquiry path is no longer productive and they wish to ponder the problem without disrupting the interview, (2) to assist in ranking of hypotheses and (3) to prevent premature closure on an obvious conclusion. When a positive finding is elicited by routine questioning, hypothesis testing is again employed.

A study of nurses conducted by Gordon (1972, 1980) focused exclusively on information-seeking strategies. Basing her work on the concept attainment studies of Bruner, Austin and Goodnow (1956), Gordon described three hypothesis testing, information gathering strategies: (1) single hypothesis testing using successive scanning as a strategy characterized by testing one hypothesis at a time, discarding the hypothesis if not confirmed by the data; (2) multiple hypothesis testing using information simultaneously to test hypotheses; and (3) predictive hypothesis testing as a form of multiple-hypothesis testing which uses contextual variables to narrow down the possible hypotheses.

The sample consisted of 60 graduate students in nursing. The subjects were presented with limited clinical data (e.g. a post-surgical patient) and instructed to ask questions and explain how the information would help in deriving a diagnosis. Two tasks were presented with two information conditions — limited to a maximum of 12 questions or unlimited. It was found that all but two subjects used mixed strategies. Predictive hypothesis-testing was used primarily in the first portion of the test with a later change to single hypothesis testing. Prolonged hypothesis testing and unlimited information conditions were associated with greater inaccuracies of diagnosis.

The information obtained in the early portion of the test was used to "predict" likely problems and hence narrow later portions of the information gathering. No doubt the preliminary clinical data given to the subjects, such as the information that the patient was post-surgical, greatly limited the range of possible problems to explore, at least initially. This strategy is apparently an important one in delimiting the focus of information gathering.

Kraus (1976) examined the effects of preinformation on the characteristics subsequently identified by nurses as being descriptive of a patient. Eighty nurses were randomly assigned to one of three experimental groups: preinformation about emotional state of the patient, preinformation about the disease state, or no preinformation. After being given preinformation, the subjects were shown a short film of a patient situation. They were then given a list of characteristics associated with disease state, emotional state or neutral and asked to rate their importance and the degree of certainty the subject had that each characteristic was descriptive of the patient they saw in the film. It was found that preinformation significantly influenced the degree of certainty attributed to subsequent information but not the degree of importance. Kraus concluded that the preinformation influenced nurses to "direct their observations toward patient characteristics which were associated with the patient state described in that information." (p. 25)

While it is likely on theoretical grounds that this conclusion is accurate, only two empirical referents of "directed observation" were examined in this study — rating of confidence and of importance. Further investigation is needed on strategies used to narrow the scope of information gathering, including the influence and use of preinformation.

Tanner (1977) in her study of senior nursing students described both hypothesis-driven and "data-driven" searches. The latter strategy was comprised of asking routine general questions cued by observations of the clinical vignettes and unrelated to obvious hypotheses. For example the subject would note in the vignette that the nurse was recording the blood pressure and would ask its value. Subjects generally employed this strategy either when they had failed to generate any hypotheses or when it appeared that the hypotheses being tested were ruled out. In one situation, the more accurate diagnoses were associated with the use of general, routine questioning rather than hypothesis testing; through its use subjects were able to acquire the information necessary to avoid premature closure on an inaccurate diagnosis.

In summary, all of the studies of information seeking suggest that a clinician uses some strategy to narrow the data field. Routine general questions are typically employed until a positive finding is elicited, then data gathering becomes more focused. The risk in narrowing the data search too rapidly is premature closure on inaccurate diagnosis and/or failure to elicit data which indicate other problems. Experienced clinicians in Barrows and Bennett, Elstein, et al and Kassirer and Gorry's studies all employed a strategy to avoid such premature closure.

HYPOTHESIS ACTIVATION The research suggests strongly that early hypothesis generation is a predominant mode of diagnostic reasoning. There is further evidence that hypotheses profoundly influence the nature of the data subsequently acquired from the patient. It is of concern to educators to understand what activates these hypotheses — what strategies must students learn to retrieve the most likely hypotheses.

Elstein and associates (1978) studied eight physicians to describe the structure of initial hypotheses and the cognitive processes involved in the generation of hypotheses. The physician subjects viewed three to four films presenting the first moments in an encounter with a patient; the film was stopped periodically to ask the subject to comment on his diagnostic hypotheses and to record cues associated with the hypotheses. A total of 49 responses were evaluated. There were four characteristics of the initial hypotheses:

1. They tended to be hierarchical in organization beginning with a general diagnostic category (e.g. respiratory problem) with several subcategories (e.g. pneumonia, acute bronchitis).
2. The initial set of hypotheses usually included competing formulations, providing alternative explanations for a symptom grouping.
3. They included formulations of varying levels of specificity from organ system to specific diagnoses (e.g. respiratory problem, anemia, diabetes, GI disorder).
4. The set often included those with functional relationships to one another (e.g. anemia may be secondary to a GI disorder).

Of the four characteristics, competing formulations most consistently appeared across subjects and tasks.

The process of generating early hypotheses appeared to be direct associative retrieval, linking the presenting cue with a general diagnostic category. This process was mediated by only two consistently appearing strategies: focusing on diseases of high incidence for the patient's demographic group and attempting to think of alternative hypotheses.

The findings were, in part, corroborated in Kassirer and Gorry's (1978) study of six physicians. What they labeled as a "stringing together" of concepts in hypothesis generation may be representative of either hierarchical or functional relationships between hypotheses. They also noted the use of a third strategy mediating direct associative retrieval: the use of potential benefits of therapeutic intervention.

In sum, the generation of hypotheses is likely to be related to organization of knowledge in long-term knowledge memory and the extent to which knowledge of relationships between cues and hypotheses and among hypotheses is stored. The work of Tversky and Kahneman in the decision-theory framework suggests that the retrieval of hypotheses may be influenced by biases such as representativeness and availability of instances.

TASK ANALYSIS A major finding in virtually all studies of diagnostic reasoning is the task-specific nature of the strategies employed. It would seem intuitively obvious that the effectiveness of strategies will vary depending on the demands of the task. Hence, a fruitful line of inquiry is to define task characteristics which determine the appropriate selection of cognitive strategies.

Only one study has been conducted to systematically vary task dimensions. Elstein and associates (1978) used four fixed-order problems. Data were presented on cards with two cues per card, in a consistent order. The 22 physicians in the sample were instructed to think aloud after reading each card and to describe the hypotheses being entertained and the cues associated with them. Each problem structure was varied along two dimensions, diagnostic specificity and cue consistency. Thus cases were designed to converge on a single diagnosis, while in the other two the cues could represent more than one diagnosis. In addition, in two problems all cues were consistent with one diagnosis and in the other not all cues could be clustered.

There were significant differences on the number of cues associated with a hypotheses; these differences were due to the cue consistency dimension. An unpredicted finding was that low cue consistency led to fewer diagnostic hypotheses than high cue consistency. Two general heuristics, or strategies, emerged: (1) cues are clustered to generate hypotheses and inconsistent cues tend to be ignored, and (2) later diagnostic hypotheses are refinements or elaborations of earlier ones.

The methods employed in this study appear to be promising for further studies of task dimensions. Further research is warranted on the effects of such task characteristics as: (1) seriousness of emergent nature of presenting problem, (2) cue reliability, (3) limited number of diagnostic possibilities, (4) multiple diagnoses, (5) varying degrees of interrelationship among cues, and (6) diagnostic categories and relationships to cues which are less well-defined (as is the case for many nursing diagnoses).

CLINICIAN VARIABLES ASSOCIATED WITH CLINICAL JUDGMENT The ability to predict the probability of prospective students' success in nursing programs has occupied a large portion of the research literature in nursing education (see chapter by Grant). Investigators of clinical judgment, in a similar vein, have attempted to identify correlations of skill in clinical judgment, both for its theoretical significance, and for its practical relevance in predicting clinical performance. The predictors of clinical judgment skill have been of two main types: measures of logical reasoning and personality measures.

Four studies have investigated the relationship between logical reasoning ability and performance on components of clinical judgment. Tanner in her study of nursing students (1977) found no relationship between the Watson-Glaser Critical Thinking Appraisal (WGCTA) and any of the seven dependent measures related to clinical judgment. Matthews and Gaul (1979) studied the relationship between both undergraduate and graduate students' ability to derive nursing diagnoses from a written case study and scores on the WGCTA. Again there was no relationship. Gordon (1972) argued that the Graduate Record Examination and the Miller Analogies are measures of inferential reasoning. She examined the relationship between scores on these measures and the type of strategies used by 60 subjects in a diagnostic task. There was no significant difference between subjects with high and low inferential ability on the use of predictive strategies. Elstein and associates (1978) used three logical problems developed by Rimoldi as a measure of logical problem-solving. There were no significant correlations between logical problem-solving scores and any of the twelve dependent measures used in the high-fidelity simulations.

It is likely that the kind of reasoning tested by these standardized measures differs from that used in clinical judgment. First, as Elstein points out (1978, p. 112), the tests lack in meaningful content and are generally designed to test reasoning separate from content influence. Clinical judgment tests, on the other hand, have a strong content component. Secondly, the probabilistic nature of clinical judgment may require a different reasoning process than that required in other forms of logical problem-solving.

The predictive value of personality measures was also evaluated by Elstein and associates (1978). Four different personality measures were used; there were no consistent statistically significant relationships between any of the personality measures and any of the clinical problem-solving measures. In a study of undergraduate nursing students, Koehne-Kaplan and Tilden (1976) examined the relationship of personality type, measured by the Jungian Type survey, and clinical judgment skills, measured by a written final examination for a course on clinical judgment. There was no significant relationship between the two measures.

EDUCATIONAL APPLICATIONS OF INFORMATION-PROCESSING THEORY Several studies have been conducted to test instructional methods designed to assist students to learn the process of early hypothesis generation. The studies were based largely on the findings that students and experienced practitioners alike generate early hypotheses, despite their training to reserve judgment; it was speculated that if students could be assisted in learning to generate *appropriate* hypotheses and proceed in systematic testing of those hypotheses then many of the errors of diagnosis could be avoided.

Allal (1973) used a training model composed of two parts: having the student practice generating diagnostic hypotheses in simulated encounters and providing the student with feedback based on performance on the same encounter by experienced physicians. The feedback was of two kinds: feedback on outcomes of the physician's hypothesis generation and feedback on the processes by which the physicians derived their hypotheses. Forty-eight second year medical students were randomly assigned to one of the three treatment conditions: training with outcome feedback, training with both outcome and process feedback, no training. Both feedback groups performed significantly better than the control group on measures of problem formulation and cue classification, but not on cue utilization (cues available from film) and relationships among problem formulations. Because there were no differences on cue utilization, the differences on problem formulation can most likely *not* be attributed to failure of the control subjects to acquire sufficient cues to generate hypotheses. There were no differences between the two types of feedback.

Tanner (1977, 1981) conducted a similar study with 54 senior baccalaureate nursing students. An experimental instructional strategy using audiovisual materials was developed to teach a unit on coronary care nursing. It differed from a traditional instructional method in two respects: (1) organization of content to facilitate hypothesis generation, and (2) practice through written workbooks on generating and testing diagnostic hypotheses. The subjects were assigned to one of six treatment conditions: the experimental method, the traditional method and no instruction (control) each crossed with concurrent clinical experience or no clinical experience. Seven dependent measures were derived from performance on a videotape simulation with verbal protocol analysis. There was a significant difference between both instructional treatment groups and the control group on all measures. There was a significant method-by-experience interaction on multi-variate analysis of variance, but the univariate analysis on each of the dependent measures failed to reveal any differences. Subjects in the experimental group with concurrent clinical experience tended to generate more diagnostic hypotheses than subjects in any of the other groups, but the number of diagnostic hypotheses was only moderately correlated with accuracy.

Taylor and her associates (1978) designed a five-and-a-half week course to assist 61 first year medical students develop their ability to generate diagnostic hypotheses. The course consisted of lectures, small group discussions and several simulated patient problems for students' practice. Post-course performance was measured in a multiple choice examination and two patient management problems. Students performed satisfactorily on factual recall, cue acquisition and interpretation but performed less well on generating and revising hypotheses.

The results of these studies, together with studies of experienced clinicians (Elstein et al, 1978; Barrows and Bennett, 1972) suggest that *appropriate* hypothesis generation may be a function of level of education and experience. Allal's and Tanner's studies suggest that both medical and nursing students in later years of their education can be taught to generate more hypotheses. Presumably this process would be associated with greater precision and thoroughness of data gathering and greater diagnostic accuracy, and hence improved management decisions, yet there is no evidence to support this assumption. There is substantial evidence that thoroughness in data gathering is associated with diagnostic accuracy (Elstein, 1978). Students in their early years in nursing programs typically learn through data gathering. The point at which they begin to shift to hypothesis-testing strategies is not known; it is at this time that instruction in hypothesis-generation and systematic testing may be most fruitful in assisting the students to avoid the pitfalls of set, premature closure and misinterpretation of cues.

Two additional studies reported by Elstein et al (1978) tested effects of other instructional strategies on diagnostic reasoning processes. Sprafka (1973) conducted a study with 30 fourth year medical students on the effects of instructions concerning hypothesis generation and verbalization. Subjects were assigned to one of six treatment groups: instructions to generate hypotheses early, instructions to withhold generating hypotheses and no hypothesis generation instructions each crossed with instructions to think aloud (verbalize) while completing three PMPs or to not verbalize. Instructions about hypothesis generation had no effect on the number of hypotheses generated, thoroughness and efficiency of cue acquisition or diagnostic accuracy. However, each of these measures were significantly increased by instructions to verbalize on one of the problems. Sprafka concludes that how early a hypothesis is generated is determined more by the nature of the problem and how the diagnostician perceives the problem than it is by instructions to do so.

In Sprafka's study as in Tanner's (1977) study of nursing students there was minimal relationship between diagnostic accuracy and early hypothesis generation. Certain types of problems may be more appropriately approached with delayed hypothesis generation.

Another study conducted by Gordon (1973) was based on the proposition that clinicians should not be taught to eliminate early hypotheses and their biasing effects; instead they should be taught certain "heuristics" to use their hypotheses more effectively. Five experimental heuristics were derived from analysis of errors committed by medical students: (1) to collect only data which is related to an overall plan, (2) to hold hypotheses of specificity or generality appropriate to the data at hand, (3) to always entertain two or three competing hypotheses, (4) whenever a new hypothesis emerges, reinterpret data already collected in light of the new hypothesis, and (5) to consistently search for low-cost diagnostic tests (i.e. relatively less expensive, uncomfortable and risky) to rule out hypothesis rather than use a high-cost test which may yield a definitive diagnosis.

Thirty-two medical students were assigned to one of four treatment groups: half were trained to use the experimental heuristics and half were asked to generate and employ a set of personal heuristics they had found useful in past diagnostic tasks. Half of each of these groups were systematically prompted to use the heuristics and half were not. Performance on a simulation was measured on scope of early hypotheses, number of critical findings elicited, cost of diagnostic work-up and accuracy of the diagnosis. There were no significant differences between any of the treatment groups on univariate analysis. Multivariate analysis did reveal a significant main effect due to heuristic training. This was interpreted as modest support for teaching students the use of heuristics in hypothesis guided search.

Toward a Synthesis of Perspectives

Research on clinical judgment has been conducted within two divergent theoretical perspectives, using different methods and designed to address different questions. Studies within the decision-theory perspective use mathematical models to prescribe optimal clinical judgment processes. Studies within the information processing theory rely on introspective verbal accounts to describe the actual clinical judgment processes employed.

Despite these differing viewpoints, the two perspectives converge on several important elements. Both agree that clinical judgment is a complex process requiring consideration of probabilistic relationships between cues and diagnoses and between diagnosis and management strategies. The decision-theory studies have found that the human judge performs less than optimally as prescribed by any mathematical model. Information-processing studies have implicitly sought to find explanations for the differences. Studies within both perspectives are analytic, describing isolated components of the judgment process. Both generally agree that the clinical judgment process is comprised of selecting alternatives, gathering information to reduce uncertainty about the alternatives, selecting the most likely diagnosis or the optimal management plan.

It can be concluded from the non-nursing literature, that the clinical judge uses strategies to adapt his/her limited resources to the demands of the task environment. The diagnostic process employed by physicians *under simulated conditions* is comprised of the generation and testing of diagnostic hypotheses. Several strategies, as well as biases, influence which hypotheses are activated and how they are evaluated. There have been no conclusive studies on the strategies used in making medical management decisions.

Similarly there have been no conclusive studies examining the influence of categories of variables (contextual, task, clinician or risk/benefit) on the clinical judgment process. There have been no studies examining contextual variables. An analysis of task complexity was a significant theoretical contribution in decision-theory paradigm but, to date, there has been no study within this framework which systematically varies task complexity. Almost every study conducted within the information processing paradigm has concluded that the cognitive strategies employed by the clinician are task specific. The task characteristics which influence the judgment process may be those related to complexity and/or those related to the clinician's knowledge of content required for the task. Only one study within the information processing paradigm has explored task characteristics. None have examined the extent to which differences between novice and expert performance, or differences in within-group or within-individual performance can be attributed to variations in relevant knowledge.

The search for clinician variables (logical reasoning ability and personality profiles) associated with the judgment process has been fruitless. This is likely to continue to be the case until the construct of clinical judgment is better defined and the processes employed are better understood; then predictors of clinical judgment performance can be more reasonably identified.

Risk/benefit variables are an inherent component of decision-theory, particularly utility theory. Research within this paradigm has suggested that the human judge performs suboptimally when compared with the statistical model. There has been no investigation specifically directed toward identifying the cognitive strategies employed when risk/benefit factors are systematically varied. In summary, while general strategies of clinical judgment, particularly diagnostic reasoning, have been described, there is little information about how these strategies will differ when other variables are considered.

The studies on clinical judgment in nursing are summarized in Table 1. While components of the clinical judgment process have been examined in isolated studies, only the series of studies conducted by Hammond and associates have attempted a comprehensive examination of inference in nursing. The potential for significant contributions in all areas of the clinical judgment process is clear — in testing the applicability of the generally accepted model of diagnostic reasoning to nursing, and analyzing the relationship between all classes of variables to the judgment process.

TABLE 1

Summary of Nursing Studies by Classification and Author

	Hammond et al (1966a)	Hammond et al (1966b)	Hammond et al (1966c)	Hammond et al (1967)	Grier (1976)	Aspinall (1977)	Gordon (1972, 1980)	Matthews & Gaul (1979)	Koehne-Kaplan & Tilden (1976)	Tanner (1977, 1981)	Kraus (1976)
I. Theoretical Perspective											
Decision Theory	X	X	X	X	X	X					
Information Processing Theory							X	X	NA	X	X
II. Component of Process											
Use of Information and Information Seeking	X	X	X				X	X	NA	X	X
Diagnosis						X	X	X		X	
Management		X		X							
III. Variables											
Contextual											
Task											
Clinician							X	X	X	X	
Risk/Benefit				X							
IV. Instructional Methods						X				X	

The analytic approaches embodied in both theoretical perspectives, and particularly the use of simulation, are constrained in their capacity to lead to an overall or gestalt view of the judgment process — as it is actually used in practice. A promising approach to the study of clinical judgment has been recently introduced to nursing by Benner. Although the full technical report of her work was unavailable at the time of this writing, some important considerations can be drawn from her published synopsis. (Benner and Wrubel, 1982).

Benner and Wrubel studied the acquisition of skilled knowledge by obtaining reports of critical incidents from expert nurses. They provide examples of clinical judgment incidents which support the notion that expert judgment derives from a grasp of the whole situation — a qualitative or perceptual assessment based on a combination of "the senses of touch, smell and sight and on the interpretation of a patient's physical, verbal and behavioral express" (p. 12). These perceptual and holistic judgments differ from objective, measurable judgments such as those elicited through use of simulation. The expert clinical judge is characterized by the ability to switch with facility from a deliberative, systematic analysis of clinical data to rapid recognition of a whole clinical situation. The beginner, possessing theoretical knowledge but lacking in practical knowledge, must use each of their sensory abilities separately, carefully analyzing and weighing each cue.

Benner and Wrubel's approach to the study of clinical judgment derives from a phenomenological perspective and is responsive to criticism of artificial intelligence issued by Dreyfus (1979). Dreyfus argues that subjecting problem-solving processes to the precise analysis required for developing computer programs completely ignores capabilities which characterize human performance. For example, awareness of peripheral information, "the fringes of consciousness", may profoundly influence how the human judge structures the problem, yet such awareness cannot be described in the verbal protocols nor used by a computer. Insight, another phenomenon documented by early problem-solving investigations, is poorly addressed in the information processing approaches. In addition, the human problem-solver can tolerate ambiguity in the situation without having to transform the situation to a context-free, precise description; verbal protocol analysis fails to capture this ability.

Thus, the approach to the study of clinical judgment within the phenomenological perspective differs greatly from that prescribed by the more analytic theories of decision making and information process. The study of expert judgment within this perspective requires examination of performance in the naturalistic environment and an exploration with the clinician of contextual factors associated with the judgment process. The approach holds potential for understanding the judgment skills of the expert in a way that may not be adequately described by the more analytic methods.

Implications for Nursing Education

The following implications are based on three major assumptions: (1) the cognitive strategies of clinical judgment which have been described through use of simulations and verbal protocol analysis are representative of those used in practice, (2) the cognitive strategies used by novice and expert physicians are not dissimilar to those used by novice and expert nurses, even though the content may differ, (3) strategies used by experts are those adopted by novices and the documented variations in performance are related to differences in level of knowledge needed to complete the task.

The development of clinical judgment skill is a combination of: (1) skill acquisition in data gathering including interviewing and physical examination, (2) acquisition of theoretical knowledge which can be applied in the clinical setting, and (3) learning of strategies which assist the student to optimally apply knowledge and adapt limited resources to the demands of the judgment task. At the time when students lack sufficient theoretical knowledge, early educational efforts may be best directed toward teaching comprehensive data gathering. Diagnostic accuracy is associated with thoroughness of cue acquisition: students attempting to employ the strategies used by experts without an adequate knowledge base may fail to gather relevant data. Later educational efforts may be best directed toward assisting students to understand and use systematically several heuristics associated with expert performance including those suggested by Gordon (1973).

Consideration of competing alternatives is a central component of all theories of clinical judgment. In diagnosis, the generation of early diagnostic hypothesis is a critical determinant of the data acquired during the diagnostic work-up and is thus indirectly related to diagnostic accuracy. The content and specificity of early hypotheses is probably related to organization of knowledge in long-term memory.

In medicine the hierarchical organization of medical knowledge, from organ systems to specific disease entities and associated cues, facilitates retrieval of diagnostic hypotheses. Efforts should be directed to assist students in organizing nursing knowledge in such a way that hypotheses can be easily activated. This may take the form of a conceptual framework. It is critical that the framework be sufficiently concrete to include specific patient problems and their associated cues as well as be sufficiently abstract to allow for a general categorization of knowledge.

Students should be assisted to search for competing explanations of clinical data and to not settle on the first diagnosis which comes to mind. Students may also be assisted by understanding the biases which influence their early identification of hypotheses. Although the number of diagnostic hypotheses is moderately related to diagnostic accuracy, a more critical determinant is holding the most likely diagnosis in the initial set retrieved. Similarly students should be assisted to identify alternative interventions. Introduction to basic tenets of utility theory may assist students to be more systematic in their choice among competing alternatives.

The written nursing care plan, as traditionally used, does not capture thought processes used in clinical judgment. Efforts should be directed at developing teaching methods which assist students to systematically use the strategies which they tend to adopt naturally, and to avoid their pitfalls. Because clinical judgment is a dynamic, interactive process, it is unlikely that an instrument such as the written care plan assists the student in developing such strategies; it represents the product, rather than the processes of thinking. Teaching strategies which require verbal interaction between the instructor and student are more likely to be helpful to the student in learning to acquire and use clinical data for inferences and deciding on courses of action. Written work may be useful to the extent that it assists students to make explicit the alternatives considered and the rationale for selection of alternatives.

Recommendations for Future Research

Several theoretical perspectives and methods for investigation of the processes of clinical judgment have been described in this review. The use of simulation allows for analysis of cognitive strategies at a level which may not be accessible through the methods employed in the phenomenological approach. But the resulting description is inevitably inadequate. Because of its reductionism and experimental control, critical variables which influence the judgment process may be inadvertently eliminated from study and the combined effect of multiple variables is difficult to assess with existing methods. It is recommended therefore that the study of clinical judgment in nursing use both approaches — simulation and naturalistic observation — with an eye toward a single theory which describes the development of skill in clinical judgment. Although the field of investigation in nursing clinical judgment is wide-open, the following questions are fundamental to the initial development of a model of judgment processes used in nursing:

1. To what extent does the model of diagnostic reasoning describe the strategies employed by nurses in making clinical inferences? And a corollary question: to what extent does an intuitive grasp of the whole situation used by the expert

replace systematic and analytic judgment processes? What factors determine a shift from one mode of inference to another?

2. What task characteristics are related to use of differing strategies by expert nurses? Most critical among these is the clinician's knowledge of content relevant to the task. Other task characteristics worthy of study include seriousness of presenting problem (emergency vs. non-emergency), cue reliability, cue consistency, number of plausible diagnoses or appropriate interventions, probability of risks and benefits of outcomes of interventions, and degrees of interrelationship among cues, among diagnoses and among interventions.

3. What strategies are used by novice nurses and how do these differ from those used by experts? To what extent can differing strategies be attributed to differences in level of knowledge?

4. What errors in clinical judgment strategies are committed by novice and expert nurses, independent of errors due to lack of knowledge?

5. Are there strategies which discriminate between clinical judges who accurately identify a diagnosis and appropriate plan of care and those who do not?

While these descriptive studies are being conducted, a number of teaching methods can be evaluated. Included among these are:

1. Use of formal decision methods (e.g. application of Utility Theory or decision trees) to assist students in becoming more systematic in judgment strategies.

2. Methods designed to assist students in generating and testing diagnostic hypotheses. Heuristic training, such as that employed by Gordon (1973) may be suitably tested in nursing.

3. Methods designed to assist students to attend to critical cues in a situation, including clinical rounds with experts. Although Benner and Wrubel (1982) maintain that this ability is a function of experience and may not be verbally transmitted to the novice, the approach warrants testing.

Research on clinical judgment, especially in nursing, is in its embryonic stages. The possibilities for fruitful lines of inquiry appear endless, and the above listing represents only those areas which seem to be most productive given our current state of knowledge. Clinical judgment research has profound implications for nursing education. It is an exciting time to vest creative energy in this field of investigation, to examine critically educational practices and to find ways to assist students to become astute clinical decision-makers.

This review was supported in part by a grant from the Northwest Area Foundation for an interdisciplinary study of the processes of diagnostic reasoning.

REFERENCES

Albert, D.A. Decision theory in medicine: A review and critique. *Health and Society,* 1978, *56,* 362-401.

Allal, L.K. Training of medical students in a problem-solving skill: The generation of diagnostic problem formulations. Unpublished doctoral dissertation. Michigan State University, 1973.

Aspinall, M.J. Use of a decision tree to improve accuracy of diagnosis. *Nursing Research,* May-June 1979, *28,* 182-185.

Bruner, J.S., Goodnow, J.J. and Austin, G.A. *A Study of Thinking.* New York: John Wiley and Sons, 1956.

Dreyfus, H.L. *What Computers Can't Do: The Limits of Artificial Intelligence.* New York: Harper & Row, 1979.

Dreyfus, S.E., & Dreyfus, H.L. A five-stage model of the mental activities involved in directed skill acquisition. Berkeley, California: University of California, 1980.

Ekwo, E.E. An analysis of the problem-solving process of third year medical students. In *Proceedings of the 16th Annual Conference on Research in Medical Education.* Washington, D.C. Association of American Medical Colleges, 1977.

Elstein, A.S., Kagan, N., Shulman, L.S., Jason, H., & Loupe, M.J. Method and theory in the study of medical inquiry. *Journal of Medical Education,* 1972, *47,* 85-92.

Elstein, A.S., Shulman, L.S., & Sprafka, S.A. *Medical Problem-Solving: An Analysis of Clinical Reasoning.* Cambridge, Mass.: Harvard University Press, 1978.

Ericsson, K.A., & Simon, H.A. Verbal reports as data. *Psychological Review,* 1980, *87,* 215-251.

Glaser, R. Components of a psychology of instruction: toward a science of design. *Review of Educational Research,* 1976, *46,* 1-24.

Gordon, M. Predictive strategies in diagnostic tasks. *Nursing Research,* 1980, *29,* 39-45.

Gordon, M. Strategies in Probabilistic Concept Attainment: A Study of Nursing Diagnosis. Unpublished Doctoral Dissertation. Boston College, 1972.

Gordon, M.A. Heuristic training for diagnostic problem solving among advanced medical students. Unpublished doctoral dissertation. Michigan State University, 1973.

Grier, M.R. Decision making about patient care. *Nursing Research,* 1976, *25,* 105-110.

Hammond, K.R., Hursch, C.J., & Todd, F.J. Analyzing the components of clinical inference, *Psychological Review,* 1964, *71,* 438-456.

Hammond, K.R. An approach to the study of clinical inference in nursing., Part II. A methodological approach. *Nursing Research,* Fall 1964, *13,* 315-319.

Hammond, K.R., Kelly, K.J., Schneider, R.J., & Vancini, M. Clinical inference in nursing: Analyzing cognitive tasks representative of nursing problems. *Nursing Research,* Spring 1966a, *15,* 134-138.

RESEARCH ON CLINICAL JUDGMENT

Hammond, K.R., Kelly, K.J.,Schneider, R.J., & Vancini, M. Clinical inference in nursing: Information units used. *Nursing Research,* Summer 1966b, 15, 236-243.

Hammond, K.R., Kelly, K.J., Castellan, N.J., Jr., Schneider, R.J., & Vancini, M. Clinical inference in nursing: Use of information-seeking strategies by nurses. *Nursing Research,* Fall 1966c, *15,* 330-336.

Hammond, K.R. Clinical inference in nursing: II. A psychologist's viewpoint. *Nursing Research,* Winter 1966, *15,* 27-38.

Hammond, K.R., Kelly, K.J., Schneider, R.J., & Vancini, M. Clinical inference in nursing: Revising judgments. *Nursing Research,* Winter 1967, *16,* 38-45.

Holzemer, W.L., Schleutermann, J.A., Farrand, L.L. & Miller, A.G. A validation study: Simulations as a measure of nurse practitioners' problem-solving skills. *Nursing Research,* May-June 1981, *30,* 139-144.

Kahneman and Tversky, A. Subjective probability: A judgment of representativeness. *Cognitive Psychology,* 1972, *3,* 430-454.

Kassirer, J.P., & Gorry, C.A. Clinical problem-solving: A behavioral analysis. *Annals of Internal Medicine,* 1978, *89,* 245-255.

Kelly, K.J. An approach to the study of clinical inference in nursing.; Part I. Introduction to the study of clinical inference in nursing. *Nursing Research,* Fall 1964, *13,* 314-315.

Kelly, K.J. An approach to the study of clinical inference in nursing.; Part III. Utilization of the "Lens Model" method to study the inferential process of the nurse. *Nursing Research,* Fall 1964, *13,* 319-322.

Kelly, K.J. Clinical inference in nursing.; I. A nurse's viewpoint. *Nursing Research,* Winter 1966, *15,* 23-26.

Kleinmuntz, B. Profile analysis revisited: a heuristic approach. *Journal of Counseling Psychology,* 1963, *10,* 315-324.

Kleinmuntz, B. *Formal Representation of Human Judgment.* New York: John Wiley and Sons, 1968.

Koehne-Kaplan, N.S., & Tilden, V.P. The process of clinical judgment in nursing practice: The component of personality. *Nursing Research,* 1976, *25,* 268-272.

Kozielecki, J. Psychological characteristics of probabilistic inference. *Acta Psychologica,* 1970, *34,* 480-488.

Kozielecki, J. A model for diagnostic problem solving. *Acta Psychologica,* 1972, *36,* 370-380.

Kraus, V.L. Pre-information — its effects on nurses' description of a patient. *Journal of Nursing Education,* 1976, *15* (15), 18-26.

Ledley, R.S., & Lusted, L.B. Reasoning foundations of medical diagnosis. *Sciences,* 1959, *130,* 9-21.

Matthews, C.A., & Gaul, A.L. Nursing diagnosis from the perspective of concept attainment. *Advances in Nursing Science,* 1979, *1,* 17-26.

30

McLaughlin, F.E., Cesa, T., Johnson, H., Lemons, M., Anderson, S., Larson, P., Gibson, J., & Delucchi, K. Nurse practitioners', public health nurses', and physicians' performance on clinical simulation test: COPD. *Western Journal of Nursing Research,* 1979, *1,* 273-295.

McLaughlin, F.E., Cesa, T., Johnson, H., Lemons, M., Anderson, S., Larson, P., & Gibson, J. Nurses' and physicians' performance on clinical simulation test: Hypertension. *Research in Nursing and Health,* 1979, *2,* 61-72.

McLaughlin, F.E., Carr, J.W., & Delucchi, K.L. Selected Psychometric Properties of two clinical simulation tests. *Journal of Medical Education,* April 1980, *55,* 375-376.

McLaughlin, F.E., Carr, J.W., & Delucchi, K.L. Measurement properties of clinical simulation tests: Hypertension and chronic obstructive pulmonary disease. *Nursing Research,* January-February 1981, *30,* 5-9.

Miller, C.A. The magical number seven, plus or minus two: some limits on our capacity for processing information. *Psychological Review,* 1956, *63,* 81-97.

Neisser, U. The multiplicity of thought. In P.C. Wason & P.N. Johnson-Laird (Eds.) *Thinking and Reasoning.* Baltimore: Penguin Books, 1968.

Neufeld, V.R., Norman, G.R., Freightner, J.W., & Barrow, H.S. Clinical problem-solving by medical students: A cross sectional and longitudinal analysis. *Medical Education,* 1981, *15,* 315-322.

Newell, A., Shaw, J.D., & Simon, H.A. Elements of a theory of human problem-solving. *Psychological Review,* 1958, *65,* 151-166.

Newell, A., Simon, H.A. *Human Problem Solving.* Englewood Cliffs, N.J.: Prentice-Hall, 1972.

Nisbett, R.E., & Wilson, T.D. Telling more than we know: verbal reports as data. *Psychological Review,* 1977, *84,* 231-259.

Savage, L.J. *The Foundations of Statistics.* New York: Wiley, 1954.

Schwartz, W.B., Gorry, G.A., Kassirer, J.P., & Essig, A. Decision Analysis and clinical judgment. *The American Journal of Medicine,* 1973, *55,* 459-472.

Schiffman, A., Cohen, S., Nowik, R., & Selinger, D. Initial diagnostic hypothesis: Factors which may distort physician's judgment. *Organizational Behavior and Human Performance,* 1978, *21,* 305-315.

Simon, H.A. Information processing theory of human problem solving. In Estes, W.K. (Ed) *Handbook of Cognitive Process Volume 5: Human Information Processing.* Hillsdale, N.J.: Laonimc Earlbaum Associates, 1978.

Slovic, P., & Lichtenstein, S. Comparison of bayesian and regression approaches to the study of information processing in judgment. *Organizational Behavior and Human Performance,* 1971, *6,* 649-744.

Sprafka, S.A. The effects of hypothesis generation and verbalization on certain aspects of medical problem solving. Unpublished doctoral dissertation. Michigan State University, 1973.

Tanner, C.A. Instruction in the diagnostic process: An experimental study. In Kim, M.J., & Moritz, D. (Ed.) *Proceedings of the Third and Fourth National Conferences on Classification of Nursing Diagnoses,* New York: McGraw Hill, 1981.

Tanner, C.A. The effect of hypothesis generation as an instructional method on the diagnostic processes of senior baccalaureate nursing students. Unpublished doctoral dissertation. University of Colorado, 1977.

Tanner, C.A. Testing for process: simulation and other alternative modes of evaluation. In *Developing Tests to Evaluate Performance in Baccalaureate Nursing Students.* NLN Publications, 1979.

Taylor, P.J., Harasym, P.H., & Laurenson, R.D. Introducing first year medical students to early diagnostic hypotheses. *Journal of Medical Education,* 1978, *53,* 402-409.

Taba, H., & Elzey, F.F. Teaching strategies and thought processes. *Teachers College Record,* 1964, *65,* 524-534.

Tversky, A., & Kahneman, D. Judgment under uncertainty: Heuristics and Biases. *Science,* 1974, *185,* 1124-1131.

Tversky, A., & Kahneman, D. Availability: A heuristic for judging frequency and probability. *Cognitive Psychology,* 1973, *5,* 207-232.

Tversky, A., & Kahneman, D. The framing of decisions and the psychology of choice. *Science,* 1981, *211,* 453-458.

Wortman, P.M. Medical diagnosis: an information processing approach. *Computers and Biomedical Research,* 1972, *5,* 315-318.

Chapter Two:
Professional Socialization
of the Registered Nurse

Chapter Two:
Professional Socialization
of the Registered Nurse

Annita B. Watson, R.N., D.N.S.

INTRODUCTION

Nursing is currently undergoing dynamic reconsideration of itself and its social role. Conflicts in definition of and preparation for the nursing role have been brought sharply into focus with the 1978 American Nurses' Association's Entry Into Practice Resolution which designated baccalaureate education as the minimum educational preparation for entry into professional nursing practice. There is, at last, with the adoption of the National League for Nursing (NLN) Board of Directors' Position Statement (1982) consensus as to the level of education necessary for professional practice. There is agreement by the professional organizations that baccalaureate education is the minimum education necessary for professional nursing practice. There is not, however, agreement that there should be "one" pathway of formal education. Nor is there agreement as to a differentiation of function or performance according to type of educational preparation.

Currently there are three distinct types of educational programs which prepare nurses for licensure: diploma, associate degree, and baccalaureate programs. According to the state nursing practice acts, graduates of all three prelicensure programs are accorded the title of "registered nurse," and legally are held accountable for having equivalent minimal nursing knowledge. Members of the nursing profession now are considering the feasibility of differentiated licensure based upon educational background. The proposed change is to reorganize nursing into two groups: professional nurses and technical nurses (Dennis & Janken, 1979). Under this plan, the title of professional nurse would be reserved for graduates of baccalaureate programs while diploma and associate degree graduates would be classified as technical nurses.

The plan to differentiate licensure according to educational background, such as professional and technical nurses, is controversial. Proponents of this position assert that a distinction can and should be made between professional and technical nursing practice, that students of respective programs have been educated and socialized to perform differently. Generally, the plan is receiving strong support within nursing but there are many who oppose the plan. The prevailing argument cited by the opposition is that there is a lack of research evidence to support the idea that baccalaureate degree graduates practice nursing any differently than diploma or associate degree graduates (Dennis & Janken, 1979). Proponents of this position contend that unless it can be demonstrated that graduates from different types of education programs practice nursing differently, no distinction by licensure should be made between them. An issue of paramount importance to this controversy is whether or not the type of educational preparation has a significant effect on nursing performance.

Three types of pre-licensure programs still exist. Despite the reduction in number, diploma schools remain a viable alternative for students seeking education in nursing. Ehrat (1981) wrote:

> Perhaps because the three nursing educational tracks — diploma, associate degree, and bachelor degree — evolved at different times for different reasons, there was no definite articulation of the differences between and among graduates. (p. 489)

Graduates of all three types of nursing education programs were and are expected to pass the same state board examination, which addresses the minimum competency required for safe nursing practice. There are no other universal certification processes that would further delineate practitioner competencies. Nursing is faced with the commonly accepted view that a "nurse is a nurse is a nurse" regardless of preparation.

Educators have sought and are continually seeking to identify and measure distinguishing characteristics among graduates. Both descriptive literature and research literature support the contention that differences exist. Yet, employers have made little attempt to distinguish among the practitioners and tend, therefore, to use new graduates of the three types of academic programs interchangeably. There is evidence that the employers tend to rate graduates' performance differently. However, despite this recognition, they do not reward graduates by assignment of functions and responsibilities according to type and length of educational preparation.

The three basic types of programs (diploma, associate degree, baccalaureate degree) are developed around occupational expectations and functions of its graduates. Though programs differ conceptually and structurally, each holds the expectation of professional socialization.

Professional Socialization

Professional socialization is the complex process by which a person acquires the knowledge, skills, and sense of occupational identity that are characteristic of a member of that profession. It involves the internalization of the values and norms of the group into the person's own behavior and conception (Jacox, 1973). The end product of professional socialization must be a person who has both the technical competencies and the internalized values and attitudes demanded by the profession and expected by the public at large. Professional socialization is a part of, and a responsibility of, the formal educational process (Cohen, 1981; Jacox, 1973; Rosow, 1965).

Despite the conflict surrounding the route and structure of the formalized nursing education process, there is general agreement that professional socialization does occur. Not only does it take place in formal classroom and clinical situations, but also through interaction with fellow students. Students, as well as faculty, serve as reference groups for the student in the development and acquisition of values and norms which characterize nursing.

As nursing moves toward professional status, it becomes increasingly relevant to ask: "Does professional socialization occur differently according to type of educational program completed?" and "Is there a difference in performance of graduates of these programs which can be measured and which would reflect a different socialization and learning process?" This chapter contains a review of the research on professional socialization of the registered nurse. The review includes research dealing with comparisons of both cognitive and affective outcomes of the professional socialization process among graduates of the three types of pre-licensure programs.

Review of Literature

A review of the literature indicates there are numerous studies on descriptive characteristics of nursing performance according to type of educational preparation. There is also evidence that cognitive performance relates to educational programs and attitudes toward practice among nurses. The review of literature is therefore divided into two main sections: (a) a brief section which reports on descriptive characteristics of performance, and (b) a section which reviews studies that have investigated differences in cognitive skills and attitudes toward practice among nurses.

Descriptive Characteristics of Technical and Professional Nursing Performance

A number of differentiating characteristics between technical and professional nursing performance are commonly cited in the literature. Professional and technical nurses are described to differ in the types of nursing problems they identify (Bailey, 1966; Johnson, 1966; Schlotfeldt, 1977). Technical nurses are prepared to identify specific, concrete, frequently occurring problems. These problems are usually physiological in nature. The professional nurse is prepared to recognize a broader range of problems — abstract as well as concrete, uncommon as well as common, complex as well as more specific, and psychosocial as well as physiological in nature. A second characteristic commonly cited is problem solving capacity (Bailey, 1966; Johnson, 1966; Schlotfeldt, 1977). Technical nurses are prepared to identify specific, concrete, frequently occurring problems. These problems are usually physiological in nature. The professional nurse is prepared to recognize a broader range of problems — abstract as well as concrete, uncommon as well as common, complex as well as more specific, and psychosocial as well as physiological in nature. A second characteristic commonly cited is problem solving capacity (Bailey, 1966; Johnson, 1966; Schlotfeldt, 1977; Tschudin, 1964). Technical nurses are described as having at their command a wide range of established interventions which can be used to solve problems. In contrast, professional nurses in addition to known, effective interventions are able to modify and innovate ways of solving problems.

Other distinguishing characteristics which illustrate a difference is the varying ability of students to assess the current nursing knowledge base and a difference in their leadership abilities. Technical nurses are expected to have at their command a good grasp of relevant and current nursing knowledge, whereas professional nurses are expected to go beyond this by recognizing gaps in the knowledge base currently in use and appreciating the value of research in advancing nursing science. According to Manthey (1967), technical nurses are depicted as having a leadership role but in general this role is restricted to the technical aspects of nursing care. In contrast, professional nurses are portrayed as assuming a leadership role in nursing's collaboration with other health care disciplines.

Observations by nursing administrators support findings in the literature of differences in performance of technical and professional nurses. Rotkovitch (1976) and Beverly and Junker (1977) observed deficiencies in the abilities of associate degree nurses to assume leadership roles. Beverly and Junker (1977) commented that associate degree graduates had difficulty establishing priorities and making nursing judgments in collaborating with other health "team" members.

Another quality cited to differentiate between professional and technical nurses is their variation in attitudes toward practice (Johnson, 1966; Schlotfeldt, 1977). Professional nurses are viewed to place more value in self-directed, autonomous nursing practice than do technical nurses.

Considerable research has been done in the area of cognitive performance and attitudes toward practice among nurses from different types of programs. A review of these studies is included and is categorized by section according to cognitive performance and attitudes toward practice.

Cognitive Performance

The studies on cognitive performance have been divided conceptually into three broad areas: competency, performance, and quality of care. Within this context, the term "competency" refers to the skills a nurse has upon completion of an educational program. "Competency is an ability, talent, or skill that allows someone to do something" (McCloskey, 1981). Performance is defined as the formal exhibition of a skill, talent, or ability (Hittleman, 1976). Quality of care relates nursing performance to patient outcomes. This review examines all three areas of cognitive performance.

COMPETENCY STUDIES Studies on the effect of nursing education on practice have attempted to compare how graduates from the various educational programs identify problems and intervene in nursing care situations. These studies relied heavily on indirect measures of simulation, rating, and testing to determine the cognitive skills or competencies a nurse has upon completion of an educational program.

SIMULATIONS. Verhonick et al. (1968) developed a series of five filmed sequences portraying patient situations. They were used to compare the observational perceptions and recommended actions of 1576 registered nurses attending two national nursing conventions. The nurses' educational preparation ranged from vocational preparation with no degree to baccalaureate, master's, and doctoral degree. Nursing students were also included. The recommended actions were categorized as either supportive (those voluntary nurse actions requiring skill, knowledge, and judgment, and not requiring direction from a physician), therapeutic (those prescribed or dependent upon orders from physicians), or neither supportive nor therapeutic. The researchers observed a positive relationship, as noted by frequency of relevant observations, with academic preparation. Academic preparation was inversely related to therapeutic actions and positively related to supportive actions. The relationship of actions to educational preparation was analyzed through a tabulation of frequencies and percentages. The nurses with higher academic degrees were more likely to identify actions they could perform independently rather than actions that needed a doctor's order. These findings suggest that differently educated nurses focus on different nursing problems and that higher education yields more independent nursing actions. However, the researchers pointed out that their sample, obtained at national conventions, was probably not representative of the nursing population.

The film sequences of Verhonick et al. were used by Davis (1972; 1974) to compare nurses from different types of educational programs. Davis used the filmed sequences in 1972 to compare 20 clinical specialists with master's degrees and 20 baccalaureate degree nurses and again in 1974 to compare the 1972 data with new data obtained from 27 diploma nurses and 20 additional clinical specialists. Nurses in both studies were asked to view the films, record their observations, recommend actions, and list the reasons for their actions. The written material was assessed for number of relevant observations, number of nursing interventions, and appropriate reasons for the interventions. The conclusions of the studies paralleled those of Verhonick: the quality and quantity of care provided by clinical nurse specialists were superior to those of baccalaureate nurses, and the care provided by baccalaureate nurses was superior to that of diploma nurses. Davis also concluded that the nurses' quality of care declined if they worked several years without continuing education. In both the 1972 and 1974 study, continuing education, not experience, appeared to be the determining factor in the quality and quantity of care given by all categories of nurses. In both studies, Davis recommended that employment practices be based on continuing education rather than experience.

Findings in each study support the contention that differently educated nurses focus on different problems and that higher education yields more independent nursing actions. There is no confirmation, however, that nurses' responses to a filmed patient situation is a true representation of their responses to a real patient.

RATINGS. Some studies have relied on ratings and tests to determine differences in competency according to type of educational preparation. The term "competency" here again refers to the skills a nurse has upon completion of an educational program.

One way to compare the competencies of program graduates is to compare the perceptions of faculty. Moore (1967) asked faculty of diploma, associate, and baccalaureate degree programs to rate 32 questionnaire items as to (a) their importance for graduates of a given program and (b) the extent to which the rater had seen such behavior in graduates of a given program. The items described qualities of leadership, judgment, and responsibility. All of them were considered more important and were seen more often in baccalaureate graduates by faculty of all three programs.

Chamings and Treevan (1979) asked nursing deans and directors of 100 baccalaureate degree and 100 associate degree programs to rate their graduates on expected competencies on an 80-item questionnaire. Useful questionnaires were retrieved from 57% of baccalaureate degree deans and 50% of associate degree directors. The authors concluded that the expectations for graduates of the baccalaureate degree programs are higher but are not clearly different.

Bullough and Sparks (1975) conducted a questionnaire survey of 201 associate degree senior students and 192 baccalaureate degree students in Los Angeles. They found that associate degree students are more cure-oriented. The authors pointed out that this care-cure dichotomy frequently prevents the upward mobility of the associate degree nurse — she is seen as different than the baccalaureate degree nurse and is frequently forced to repeat nursing content, presumably with a different emphasis.

A different approach was chosen by Watson (1981) in her research dealing with the differentiation of professional and technical function in nursing. She developed her study from a theoretical framework of professional and technical characteristics in society, classification systems of the United States Department of Labor, and concepts derived from engineering literature regarding professional and technical functions. Watson used the survey method to determine expectations of functions from both associate degree and baccalaureate degree nursing programs and graduates. A sample of 123 bachelor's degree and 134 associate degree programs and 216 bachelor's degree and 213 associate degree graduates located in 193 United States hospitals were randomly selected to participate in the study.

According to the percentage analysis of current functions, bachelor's and associate degree programs and their graduates expect the respective graduates to perform all technical and various professional functions. According to the determination of most characteristic functions, bachelor's degree programs identified professional and associate degree programs identified technical functions. Watson also found an inverse relationship of professional functions of the bachelor's degree in proportion to hospital size."The larger the hospital, the more likely it is the graduate will function as a technician" (Watson, 1981, p. 571-B).

Dennis and Janken (1979) concluded from their review of the literature that diploma and associate degree nurses are more likely to focus on basic skills and technical care delivery, while baccalaureate nurses are more likely to focus on activities requiring leadership, psychosocial skills, and problem solving. McCloskey (1981) supported these conclusions based on her review of the literature.

TESTS.   Mandrillo (1970) developed an objective, multiple-choice test to assess cognitive skills in relating scientific knowledge to patient problems. The test was administered to 155 graduating baccalaureate degree students and 106 graduating associate degree students enrolled in five universities and four colleges in New York City. Although Mandrillo's instrument had a reported reliability of .87, validity was not ascertained. The graduating baccalaureate students were found to score significantly higher than the associate degree students on cognitive abilities and recall of knowledge, as well as on skills in applying knowledge to four patient problems.

Additional attempts have been made by Gray et al. (1977) and Scoloveno (1981) to differentiate between technical and professional nursing. Gray et al. (1977) used open-ended short essay questions based on clinical situations to compare the responses of 22 graduating associate degree and 22 graduating baccalaureate students. Responses to the questions were coded as being expected of: all nurses, only technically prepared nurses, or only professionally prepared nurses. Some differences were found in the following aspects of nursing care: technical skills, leadership, support given to patients and their families, interviews of patients for assessment purposes, nursing actions in structured situations, and nursing actions following observations. Baccalaureate students initiated non-prescribed nursing actions and anticipated long-term needs more often than associate degree nurses.

The test's reliability and validity are not sufficiently addressed in the study report.

In 1981, Scoloveno conducted a study to ascertain whether differences exist in the problem solving ability of senior students from baccalaureate, associate degree, and hospital-based nursing programs. The Revised Nursing Process Utilization Inventory (reported reliability of .85) and the Watson-Glaser Critical Thinking Appraisal were used to measure the participants' problem solving and critical thinking abilities. The study consisted of 90 baccalaureate, 93 associate degree, and 97 hospital-based students in nine nursing programs. Statistical analysis of the data revealed that: (a) baccalaureate students obtained significantly higher scores beyond the .01 level of confidence on both simulated nursing situation tests in the Revised Nursing Process Utilization Inventory when compared to associate degree and hospital-based nursing students; (b) baccalaureate students obtained significantly higher scores $p < .01$ on the Watson-Glaser Critical Thinking Appraisal than did associate degree or hospital-based students; (c) the mean scores of associate degree and hospital-based students were not significantly different on the test reflecting a primary health-care situation, and (d) associate degree students obtained significantly higher scores beyond the .01 level of confidence than did hospital-based students on the simulated acute and chronic care situation in the Revised Nursing Process Utilization Inventory. Scoloveno concluded that baccalaureate nursing students appear to have a better foundation in general education and nursing theory.

Polifroni (1981) analyzed problem solving abilities of senior nursing students in preservice and inservice baccalaureate programs. The study sample included 90 students from three preservice, generic, programs, 85 students from three generic baccalaureate programs for inservice (R.N.) students, and 83 students from three upper division baccalaureate programs designed specifically for inservice (R.N.) students. Three instruments were used to measure the dependent variable of problem solving ability, and the four covariates of age, aptitude, years of post-secondary education, and years of prior health-related work experience: the Revised Background Questionnaire, the Watson-Glaser Critical Thinking Appraisal, and the Revised Process Utilization Inventory. The investigator found that the generic baccalaureate preservice and inservice students scored significantly higher on the Watson-Glaser Critical Thinking Appraisal Test and on both tests of the Nursing Process Utilization Inventory than did the inservice students in the upper division baccalaureate programs. Polifroni concluded that graduates of a generic baccalaureate nursing program are superior in problem solving skills to graduates of an upper division baccalaureate program limited to inservice students. "Therefore, this study served to add to the literature supporting the generic baccalaureate degree as a means of professionalizing nursing and nursing education" (p. 1395 B).

These studies attempt to describe and compare a nurse's competence and skills upon graduation from different types of educational programs. It is not known, however, whether competence in school is equivalent to competence on the job. A review of studies of competencies on the job or performance (McCloskey, 1981) follows.

PERFORMANCE STUDIES The majority of performance studies focus on ratings by others, directors of nursing and head nurses, or the nurses themselves. Performance studies using ratings by directors of nursing are subject to the same criticism as the competency studies using ratings by educators. Most of the ratings are not done by direct observation, but depend upon the directors' perceptions of a group of people with a particular educational background (McCloskey, 1981). The response of the directors and educators may be biased by their own educational background and the type of nurses they encounter.

RATINGS BY OTHERS. Waters et al. (1972) combined several types of performance ratings. These researchers assessed the perceptions of head nurses and directors of nursing of professional and technical nurses and observed and interviewed nurses while they practiced in the clinical setting. The sample included 12 directors of nursing, 22 head nurses, 24 associate degree nurses, and 24 baccalaureate degree nurses. A critical incident technique was used to elicit differences in the decision making process. Data were categorized according to three areas: the decision making process, scope of practice, and attitude toward practice. The associate degree nurses tended to identify only problems which were concrete and specific, and physiological in nature. Their nursing actions tended to have predictable outcomes. In contrast, the baccalaureate degree nurse considered patients' psychological and social needs. Six of the 24 baccalaureate degree graduates were also more self-directed and extended their practice beyond the standardized approach. It was also observed that the majority of baccalaureate nurses who demonstrated professional behavior came from the same hospital which had a high proportion of baccalaureate nurses on staff.

Despite methodological problems — small sample size, generalizations drawn from two critical incidents to a nurse's entire practice, confusing answers from head nurses, and a possibly biased rating from directors — Waters and her colleagues believed that the study supported the commonly held belief that professional nursing practice is a function of the setting.

Cicatiello et al. (1974) described a limited survey with a different respondent population. Eighteen nursing directors were queried about their opinions of associate degree nurses. The majority of the respondents said that associate degree nurses functioned in their hospitals as team leaders or team members. Most of the directors agreed that knowledge of nursing theory was the associate degree graduate's greatest strength. Weaknesses cited were: insufficient clinical experience to translate theory into action, lack of pharmacological knowledge, inability to handle evening and night duty, and lack of organizational and decision making skills.

Howell (1978) mailed a questionnaire to the directors of nursing of 86 hospitals and had them rank order their perception of the performance of new graduates from associate degree, diploma, and baccalaureate degree programs. The directors gave lower rankings to the associate degree nurse. Directors of small hospitals ranked the diploma nurse as more valuable whereas directors of large hospitals considered the baccalaureate degree nurse more valuable. Nearly all directors believed that the differences in initial capabilities decreased with time. Methodological problems of the study were: a response rate of 58%, no reliability or validity of the questionnaire, and no statistical analysis of the data.

Similarly, Zarett (1980) asked the directors of nursing in 323 hospitals to rate performance of graduates of associate degree, diploma, and baccalaureate degree programs on eleven nursing activities. Forty-eight per cent of useful questionnaires were returned. The directors rated diploma graduates significantly higher on six of the eleven activities, the same in three activities, and lower in only two activities. Zarett stated that the tool was assessed for content validity and that test reliability was ascertained but did not state the method or results. She did not control for educational background of the directors.

Welches, Dixon and Stanford (1979) obtained head nurse ratings on 650 nurses in the San Francisco Bay area. They compared the ratings with information collected from the 650 nurses on numerous variables which were then clustered in 12 groups. The variable clusters which correlated with the head nurse ratings were: (a) age and experience, (b) intelligence, sensitivity, and flexibility; (c) job satisfaction and opportunity for professional growth; (d) perception of self-performance; (e) social image; and (f) leadership potential and capacity for status. The educational background of the nurse did not correlate with head nurse ratings.

In 1975, Kramer and Schmalenberg conducted an experimental study of reality shock, the shock that new graduates experience when they move from the protected school environment to the real world of practice. In this study, reported in 1978, they introduced an inservice "bicultural" training program in eight representative American hospitals which focused primarily on interpersonal conflict resolution techniques to minimize reality shock. Nurses who were in the program were compared with nurses who were in a training program designed to simulate inservice education programs. Although the study focused on the training program itself, information about educational level and performance was analyzed. The associate degree nurses had significantly fewer above average and more below average performance ratings by head nurses than diploma or baccalaureate degree nurses. The training program was more effective in retaining both baccalaureate and associate degree graduates from different educational programs.

Petti (1975) investigated patients' as well as head nurses' ratings of diploma, associate, and baccalaureate degree nurses. Eighty-three staff nurses from ten general hospitals were evaluated by both medical-surgical patients and head nurses using the Slater Nursing Competencies Rating Scales. Patients gave consistently higher ratings than head nurses. No significant relationship was found between the educational level and average performance rating of the nurse.

RATINGS BY NURSES. Hover (1975) investigated the relationship between nurses' education and both their preferences for types of patients and their definitions of a "good nurse." A questionnaire was administered to 54 diploma nurses, 20 baccalaureate nurses, and 29 diploma nurses who were studying for their baccalaureate degree. These nurses were employed in three hospitals, had worked on inpatient units at least two months, and had obtained a diploma or a degree within the last five years. Hover found that, as education increased, nurses preferred more active patients, in contrast to ones immobilized by attachments to medical machinery, and were more interested in providing teaching and supportive care. The "good nurse" definition of baccalaureate nurses more frequently included cognitive as well as technical objectives.

Kubat (1975; 1976) administered a multiple choice test of nursing knowledge to 65 nurses by questionnaire. She concluded that younger nurses living in large communities who were employed full time, had a higher level of education, and had taken the State Board Test Pool Examination recently, were more likely to remain competent. She did not clarify the contents of the nursing competency test. The study sample was composed of one associate degree nurse, 58 diploma nurses, and only six baccalaureate degree nurses.

A nationwide study by Jacobs et al. (1978) was conducted to provide a research base for revising the State Board Test Pool Examination. The research included approximately 10,000 critical incidents (self-reports or reports about peers) provided by more than 2,000 nurses. In a secondary analysis of 1978 data, Jacobs (1980) reported that there were differences in the job competencies of diploma, associate degree, and baccalaureate degree nurses. Baccalaureate degree nurses were more often involved in incidents concerning leadership and professional responsibility, patient teaching and promotion of psychological well-being, exchanging and recording information about the patient, and planning care. While Jacobs found statistically significant differences among groups due to the large sample size, the differences may not be enough in practice to differentiate levels of performance.

Watson (1982) used Kelman's model of socialization as a framework for assessing the degree of influence an educational program has on the professional socialization of registered nurses. Two concepts were measured: attitudes of professionalism and problem identification skills. A cross-sectional survey was used to assess differences among and between graduates of five types of educational programs: diploma, associate degree, generic baccalaureate degree, and upper two and second step programs for R.N. B.S.N. completion students. A modified stratified random sampling technique was used to select a sample of 159 registered nurses who met selection criteria and agreed to participate in the study. Eighty-three percent of the sample completed the four instruments: a Demographic Survey; Hall's Occupational and Organizational Inventory; the Problem Identification Instrument; and the Benner Proficiency Scale.

Generic baccalaureate graduates held stronger attitudes toward professionalism ($p = .02$) than did diploma and associate degree graduates as measured by the Benner Real Proficiency Scale. There was no difference between performance by technical and professional graduates on problem identification skills. No differences were found in attitudes toward professionalism or problem identification skills between R.N. B.S.N. completion graduates of upper two and second step programs. A discriminant analysis confirmed the actual classification of graduates as technical or professional with 72.4% accuracy.

Watson (1982) concluded that the type of educational preparation is associated with the development of professional attitudes. She also concluded that the data suggested that baccalaureate graduates should experience less reality shock than diploma or associate degree graduates due to their higher perception of skill mastery on the Benner Proficiency Scale. The lack of significant findings on the effect of the work setting on perceptions of performance may have been due to the homogeneity of respondents and their work settings.

Three studies compared self-ratings of the nurse with ratings of others. Dyer et al. (1972) sampled 1,018 nurses from 31 Veterans Administration Hospitals and compared their self-ratings on several scales with the ratings of supervisors and head nurses. Two instruments were administered to assess the ratings of head nurses and supervisors on their perceptions of differences in performance among diploma, baccalaureate, and associate degree prepared staff nurses. Head nurses completed the Nurse Performance Descriptive Scales for Nursing Performance (DSNP). Educational level was found to be positively related to administrators' perceptions of performances on both scales. Nurses who rated highest on performance by their supervisors had a higher level of education and had done well in the more difficult academic subjects. They scored high on the California Psychological Inventory for Social Presence, Sense of Well-Being, Responsibility, Tolerance, Achievement via Conformance, and Intellectual Efficiency. Education was only one variable among many studied.

Comparative ratings were also used to assess performance predictors in Schwerian's (1977; 1978; 1979) federally-funded, national study of graduates from 151 randomly-selected, state-approved nursing schools. Schwerian compared the most promising nurses as identified by their academic achievement in nursing school with nurses not so identified on the basis of their own ratings and the ratings of their supervisors. Education was only one variable investigated. The major findings of the report include the following: Supervisors rated the performance of baccalaureate degree nurses better than diploma or associate degree nurses in Teaching/Collaboration and Planning/Evaluation; and no differences were found among baccalaureate, diploma, and associate degree nurses on Leadership, Critical Care, Interpersonal Relations, or Professional Development. The tool for data collection was carefully constructed and validated. The response rate, however, was low (30%).

Nelson's (1978) study of nurses' educational levels queried all 1974 graduates of North Dakota nursing programs and their supervisors about their perceptions of the graduates' competence in technical, communication, and administrative skills. The findings based on a 75% return of the Nurse Competence Inventory were that supervisors of baccalaureate graduates rated the graduates overall competence significantly higher ($p < .05$) than did supervisors of associate degree and diploma graduates. In the specific areas of technical, communicative, and administrative skills, supervisors of baccalaureate nursing graduates rated baccalaureate graduates' competency significantly higher ($p < .05$) than did supervisors of associate degree and diploma graduates. Nelson also found that diploma nurses rated themselves highest on technical skills, whereas baccalaureate degree graduates rated themselves highest on communicative skills. Level of education of supervisors was not controlled by the researcher. The questionnaire rating items were obtained from a review of the literature and were validated by expert opinion, but reliability data were not provided.

Although some of the performance rating studies reviewed depended upon observations of direct performance, none related nursing performance to patient outcomes. The measurement of quality care relates nursing performance to patient outcomes. Studies measuring quality of care are reviewed in the next section.

QUALITY OF CARE Two studies were reviewed: Highrighter (1969); and Haussman, Hegyvary, and Newman (1976). Only one study, Haussman, Hegyvary, and Newman (1976) revealed significant findings in associating education with level of performance. Characteristics of nurses were correlated with the quality of patient care as measured by the Rush-Medicus tool (a process measure). As part of a larger study, Haussman, Hegyvary, and Newman (1976) examined the effect the type of nursing education had on the quality of nursing performance by directly observing nurses in patient care settings. The sample included eight diploma nurses, five associate degree nurses, and 16 baccalaureate degree nurses. Diploma nurses scored higher than baccalaureate or associate degree nurses in their formulations of nursing care plans. At the same time, baccalaureate graduates scored higher than did diploma or associate degree nurses in their attention to non-physical needs and evaluation of nursing care achievements.

In spite of conflicting findings, the overall opinion of researchers represented in the studies and literature continue to support the idea that a difference exists in the quality of practice among diploma, associate degree, and baccalaureate degree prepared nurses (Dennis & Janken, 1979). It remains difficult to make a definite statement about the effect the type of nursing education has on cognitive performance in nursing care situations.

Attitudes Toward Practice

Attitudes toward practice are a reflection of the socialization process which occurs in education. Corwin, Taves, and Haas (1969) indicated that there was considerable disillusionment with nursing as a career, and that nursing students were more satisfied with nursing than were graduates. Success in practice was measured by how students and graduate practitioners were rated by their clinical instructors and supervisors. The authors attributed their findings to the fact that some characteristics such as professionalism and humanitarianism are stressed during education, while more tedious elements such as bureaucratic duties tend to be ignored. Fromm (1977), Kramer (1974), Simms (1977), Wang and Watson (1977), and Watson (1977) have elaborated on this thesis. Their studies indicate that the cause of disillusionment in nursing is rooted in the educational system and in problems in the socialization process. There is continuing controversy over the distinctions between the three types of pre-licensure programs. The controversy centers around length of program, curricula, goals, student selection, and the process of professional socialization (Cohen, 1981).

The following section explores research studies in the area of attitudes toward practice as determined by type of educational preparation. This review is presented in three main categories: attitudes of nurses; professionalism and job satisfaction; and professional orientation. Studies examine the effects of pre-licensure educational programs in the development of attitudes toward professionalism and perceptions of competencies.

ATTITUDES OF EDUCATORS AND EMPLOYERS Research on the attitudes of educators and employers and the selection process in nursing schools indicates that the three types of programs admit, educate, and graduate nurses who as groups are very much alike. Reichow and Scott (1976) surveyed employees, asking them to rate the effectiveness of graduates from different programs. Completed questionnaires were returned by 123 (74% return). Of these, 77 had experience with associate degree and baccalaureate degree graduates. Respondents ranked the different types of nurses on a scale of one to three with regard to such items as dealing with patients, performing technical procedures, adapting to new situations, expressing leadership ability, and showing initiative. In all hospitals, diploma nurses ranked highest, particularly in technical skills. Larger hospitals had a higher regard for baccalaureate graduates than did smaller ones. Both types of hospitals rated the baccalaureate nurse highest in knowledge of administrative procedures, and equal to diploma nurses in leadership and ability to learn new concepts. The associate degree graduate failed to demonstrate clear areas of strength, except for conscientiousness. Most respondents said that over time graduates of the three types of programs eventually became equal in ability.

Hogstel (1977) reported a survey which involved nurses recently graduated from two associate degree and two baccalaureate degree programs, as well as nursing directors from a variety of health agencies. A questionnaire was sent to 109 associate degree and 236 baccalaureate degree graduates in staff nurses' positions, asking them to report the extent of their performance for each of 80 activities which were categorized into five basic nursing functions. They were also asked how they perceived their preparation in each of the areas. Questionnaires were also sent to 100 randomly selected nursing directors, asking them to respond similarly. The only clear difference in functions between groups was in community health care functions. Baccalaureate graduates performed significantly more functions in the area of community health care. The baccalaureate graduates felt better prepared in this area while the associate degree graduates perceived themselves to be better prepared in physical care and technical skills. The nursing directors reported that baccalaureate graduates were better prepared at time of employment in four out of five nursing functions, but no difference was noted between types in ability to perform physical care and technical skill functions. In spite of recognized differences, the majority of directors did not differentiate between groups in orientation, beginning positions, promotions, or nursing assignments.

ATTITUDES OF NURSES Meleis and Farrel (1974) studied the attitudes of seniors from the three different types of programs to determine the quality of nursing care that could be expected from each type of graduate. Six standardized instruments were administered to a total of 188 senior students in six schools of nursing: three baccalaureate, one associate degree, and two diploma schools. Only 59% of the students asked to participate did so, and baccalaureate students had an especially low cooperation rate (46%). Minimal differences between the seniors of the different types of programs were found. The intellectual potential and the responsibility toward patients did not vary. Baccalaureate degree students showed slightly higher leadership potential. Diploma students placed highest value on research; baccalaureate students placed lowest value on research. The investigators concluded that there were more similarities among senior students in the three types of programs than many nursing educators had acknowledged.

There is evidence to suggest that nurses perceive their skills and competencies differently (Hogstel, 1977; Meleis & Farrell, 1974; Nelson, 1978; Smoyak, 1972). In general baccalaureate graduates identify themselves as stronger in communication skills than do other nurses. In contrast, the findings on administrative competencies are inconsistent.

PROFESSIONALISM AND JOB SATISFACTION Nurses' role orientation can be conducive to job satisfaction/dissatisfaction. Kramer (1974) has been instrumental in making nurses aware that a high professional role orientation can be distressing in some instances. She has pointed out that nurses educated along professional lines have placed high values on individualized, comprehensive patient care provided by well-qualified practitioners. These nurses emphasize decision making and problem solving skills. Organizations often require nurses to delegate parts of their work to lesser trained personnel and to submit to external supervision in the interest of maximum agency functioning. Consequently, conflict results when nurses who have taken on a high professional role orientation become employed in organizations which demand a division of labor. There has been indication that nurses who do not resolve this conflict are more apt to leave nursing (Dennis & Janken, 1979).

In a study of 220 baccalaureate nurses from a nationwide sample, Kramer and Baker (1971) observed that approximately one-half had left hospital nursing altogether. The highest dropout rate was among graduates with a high professional role orientation.

In light of these findings, it is of interest to determine how graduates from the different educational programs compare in professionalism and job satisfaction. Hurka (1971) studied 81 baccalaureate, 159 diploma, and 20 associate degree graduates employed in four hospitals. The professional orientation scores of baccalaureate graduates were found to be higher than diploma or associate degree graduates, but not significantly so. In addition, professional role orientation was found to be positively related to job satisfaction but not to satisfaction with nursing as a career.

Goff (1973) studied the relationship of nursing education, nurses' image of nursing, and job satisfaction. Using 875 diploma and baccalaureate nurses in the United States Air Force, the study concluded that for diploma nurses, the image of nursing in the first two years of practice does not differ from the image of nursing in subsequent years. For baccalaureate nurses, the image of nursing begins much higher than for diploma nurses, but by the beginning of the third year in practice has adjusted to the same level. Despite the differences in image of nursing, both groups of nurses had similarly lower levels of job satisfaction in the first two years of practice and higher levels thereafter.

Fogarty (1980) tested the general hypothesis that rate of employment activity between baccalaureate and diploma nurses is due to the effects of extraneous and intervening variables and not to intrinsic differences in the educational process. Mailed questionnaires from 1,475 nurses provided data on two measures of employment activity, as well as four control variables: marital status, spouse's income, presence of young children at home, and disillusionment with career. Among recent graduates, there was a negative association between possession of the baccalaureate degree and current employment. Holding the four control variables constant did not reduce this association to a near zero. Controlling for marriage, children, and disillusionment produced the opposite effect; the association between type of education and employment status actually increased. Fogarty formulated the initial conclusion that there is some intrinsic difference in the two types of education that causes diploma nurses to be more active than baccalaureate in their careers. He suggested further research be directed to examining alternative explanations for employment activity among nurses.

There is some indication that the variables, professionalism, job satisfaction, and job attrition, interact. However, it has not been shown to what extent (Dennis & Janken, 1979).

PROFESSIONAL ORIENTATION   Students' images and attitudes of nursing have been studied since the early sixties when Davis and Oleson (1964) conducted the first study. Davis and Oleson assessed identified problems in the status transition of coed to student nurse. It was found that nursing students experienced identity stress because of some of the difficulty they had in psychologically integrating the nursing student role with a concurrently emerging identity of adult woman.

PERSONALITY TRAITS.   Davis and Oleson (1965) conducted a study to determine to what extent professional education in nursing influences the students' basic attitudes toward the image of work in relation to women's roles. When asked to rank from four different attributes commonly associated with the female role, the majority of students ranked "work and career" second, after first selecting "home and family." There was no increase in the proportion doing so from entry to graduation. In 1966, Oleson and Davis again studied baccalaureate students' image of nursing. In this study, students increasingly characterized nursing and what they valued in it in terms of advanced professional images of the field. Complementary to this trend, a larger proportion of them came to reject bureaucratic images of the field, although some continued to hold on to certain lay images. Except for the students' increased endorsement of advanced professional images for both nursing and self, there was not a close correspondence between what they saw in nursing and the qualities of nursing they valued.

In studying personality changes as a result of socialization, Stromberg (1976) pointed out that the traditional female personality traits do not include independence, leadership, competence, or intellectual achievement. Therefore, changes in the student's sexual identity would be necessary to integrate the "professional nurse" and the female self-perception. As the student's sex role identity became more masculine, the student's image of nursing was more in harmony with the image advanced by the profession. The image of nursing held by baccalaureate and associate degree students was more professional than that of diploma students; however, there were no significant differences between the baccalaureate and associate degree students in this area.

PROFESSIONAL COMMITMENT.   Alutto, Hrebiniak, and Alonso (1971) also compared students from the three types of programs: measures of professional commitment, clinical specialty commitment, role conflict, interpersonal trust, and authoritarianism. They found that the students were similar in terms of their cognitive commitment to nursing. Baccalaureate students had a more professional" set of values and attitudes. For example, they expected to assume responsibility for entire tasks and many aspects of patient care, whereas students from the other types of programs were less likely to assume responsibility for tasks and numerous aspects of patient care. The investigators also found that the baccalaureate nurse did not demonstrate an ability to cope with confrontation between bureaucratic and professional ideals.

Cohen (1981) concluded that these findings indicate that although trust and compliance may be easier for the baccalaureate students, there is no evidence that constructive rebellion is encouraged in baccalaureate programs any more than it is in the other two programs. "B.S.N. practitioners play their roles as programmed by the socializers" (Cohen, 1981, p. 76). They are told they will become uncomfortable upon graduation and experience role conflict. Upon graduation, they do, in fact, experience role conflict. Their response is not to rebel. According to Corwin, Taves, and Haas (1961), they internalize another set of values, eventually become disillusioned, or they leave the field. In contrast, diploma students are not likely to identify with the faculty and will not show corresponding trust. They learn to exhibit the appropriate attitudes that allow them to fit into the hospital setting and survive. Diploma nurses express lower professional and service conceptions of role than diploma students do, suggesting that these are maintained. Diploma students experience less reality shock and remain in hospital nursing. They are not as indoctrinated by the faculty as are baccalaureate nursing students (Corwin, Taves, & Haas, 1961).

These studies on professional commitment show little change from studies conducted by Dustan (1964) and Ventura (1976). Dustan's and Ventura's studies indicated few differences in personality traits, intellectual qualities, professional attitudes, or the image of nursing held by the graduates of the different programs.

ROLE ORIENTATION.   Research on changes in attitudes and values over time indicates that some changes do occur. Sharp and Anderson (1972) in their exploration of nursing students' descriptions of the personality characteristics of the ideal nurse found that differences between seniors and freshmen existed. The students' descriptions became progressively similar to the faculty's descriptions as the students progressed in their program. On the test as a whole, however, seniors differed significantly from faculty. Fewer graduating students than entering students agreed on an image of nursing. As freshmen, they apparently shared strong and consistent images of the role promoted by public culture.

In 1968, Siegel assessed the degree professional socialization occurred in two programs. Investigation was limited to two baccalaureate programs. Seniors' perceptions of nursing and related values were found to correspond closely with those of faculty members. Students assigned greater personal importance to advanced professional characteristics at later stages in both programs but did not typically attribute these characteristics to their picture of nursing.

May and Ilardi (1970) used the Allport-Vernon-Lindzey Study of Values to investigate value changes among 41 baccalaureate nursing students during their educational experience. Findings suggest that there was a significant decrease in mean scores on the theoretical and religious value scale and an increase in mean scores on the aesthetic and political value scale. Few other changes were found.

Knox (1971) studied the formation of nurse role conceptions in baccalaureate students. Two groups of subjects were chosen from six accredited programs for comparative study. Data were collected from 235 neophyte students who were completing the first year of the nursing major and 153 senior students. The results indicated that senior students had significantly higher professional conceptions of the role of the nurse, and significantly lower bureaucratic conceptions than the neophytes. There was no significant difference between their service role conceptions, both groups expressing high humanitarian values. The majority of students identified a faculty member or nurse practitioner as a role model. A difference was noted between the professional role conception of neophytes who specified different role models; the highest professional conception was reported by neophytes with instructor role models. It was concluded that faculty have a major influence on the students' formation of nurse role conceptions. The study suggests that students acquire professional conceptions, sustain service conceptions, and reject bureaucratic conceptions during the school experience.

In 1972, Davis studied the effects of anticipatory socialization on role formation. Role conceptions, role deprivations, and adaptive role strategies were investigated to determine differences between graduating students, faculty members, and students and faculty in associate and baccalaureate degree programs. Differences between faculties and between faculty and students within each type of program were similarly investigated. Associate degree students had significantly higher means than baccalaureate students on bureaucratic role conceptions and bureaucratic response strategies. Baccalaureate degree students had significantly higher means on professional and service role conceptions and on bureaucratic, professional, and service role deprivation. Faculty of the different programs responded similarly. It was concluded that differences between students within a program were as great as, if not greater than, differences between students from the two types of programs.

Tetreault (1976) examined the correlation between professional attitudes and selected situational and demographic factors of baccalaureate nursing students. Professional attitudes were found to be highest for students 24 to 26 years of age, who saw nursing as highly positive and highly active, who had the largest number of formal and informal nursing experiences, and whose teachers were seen as trustworthy and professional. Werner (1973) also examined the influence teachers have on the students in terms of professional socialization, and concluded that anything a student learns about the faculty, good or bad, stands a chance of being incorporated into that student's value system.

Brown, Swift, and Oberman (1974) replicated the Davis and Oleson (1964) study. Their findings led support to the assumptions of Davis and Oleson that collegiate nursing students are recruited from a common pool of applicants, similar in social background, aspirations, and beliefs. These students shared the humanistic and professional views, rather than the bureaucratic views expressed by students in the earlier study.

Eller (1976) investigated the role orientation toward professional nursing of senior students in associate degree, diploma, and baccalaureate nursing education programs just prior to graduation. Data were obtained on attitudes toward nursing by means of a professionalization scale (the scale was not identified) administered to 358 graduating students: 127 associate degree, 100 diploma, and 131 baccalaureate nursing students. Findings indicated that the attitudes of all the senior nursing students moved slightly toward a professional orientation. However, the attitudes of the students in the three programs differed significantly. The baccalaureate students were more professionally-oriented toward nursing than were associate degree and diploma students.

Symbolic interactionist theory formed the framework for a study completed by Thomas (1978). The purpose of the study was to determine whether students from four different types of programs held different professional orientations and role conceptions as a result of the professional socialization process. The Nurses' Professional Orientation Scale (NPOS), with reliability of .89 and construct validity, was administered to a sample of 178 senior nursing students and 92 faculty. The sample represented four different types of nursing programs: associate degree, diploma, generic baccalaureate, and baccalaureate for registered nurses. Professional orientation scores did not differ significantly from program to program. The only significant differences in traditional/nontraditional role conceptions occurred between the traditionally-oriented associate degree and diploma programs and the baccalaureate program for registered nurses, which held the most nontraditional orientation.

The research to date gives some indication that type of education affects the way in which nurses perceive their own competencies. In general, baccalaureate graduates of pre-licensure programs tend to score higher than other nurses on measures of professionalism.

Summary

Numerous studies have been conducted in the area of cognitive performance and attitudes toward practice among nurses from different types of programs. Studies on cognitive performance have been executed in the areas of competency, performance, and quality of care. Within the area of competency (skills a nurse has upon completion of an educational program), studies relied heavily on inherent measures of simulation, ratings, and tests. Findings in each simulation study reviewed supported the contention that differently educated nurses focus on different problems and that higher education yields more independent nursing actions. The studies which focused on ratings also revealed differences in the focus of care according to level of educational preparation. Many of these studies, however, suffered from methodological weaknesses as did many of the studies using tests to determine differences.

Although some conclusive evidence was found which differentiated competencies among nurses upon graduation, it was not determined whether competence in school was equivalent to competence on the job. Performance studies in the form of ratings by others and self were reviewed to determine if on-the-job performance differences existed. Most of the ratings which were reviewed were not done by direct observation. Many of the studies were dependent upon employers' perceptions about a group of people with a particular educational background, and therefore may reflect a biased response. Differences in perception of performance were also documented. However, none of the studies related nursing performance to patient outcomes. Three studies did attempt to correlate patient care outcomes with nurse characteristics.

The review of cognitive performance revealed conflicting findings. The overall opinion of researchers represented, however, continued to support the premise that a difference exists in the performance among graduates of different types of educational programs.

Research on attitudes toward practice suggested that nurses perceive their skills and competencies differently. Baccalaureate graduates tended to identify themselves as stronger in communication skills than did other nurses. There was also some indication that the variables of professionalism, job satisfaction, and job attrition interact. However, the extent has not been demonstrated. Few differences in personality traits, intellectual qualities, professional attitudes, or the image of nursing held by the graduates of the different programs were documented in the research which was reviewed.

In general, the research to date can be interpreted as giving some indication that type of education affects the way in which nurses perceive their own role and competencies. Baccalaureate graduates of pre-licensure programs tended to score higher than other nurses on measures of professionalism.

The research evidence is inconclusive. The questions remain: "Does professional socialization occur differently according to type of educational program completed?" and "Is there a difference in performance of graduate of these programs which can be measured and which would reflect a different socialization and learning process?"

Implications For Nursing Education

Thus far the studies aimed at demonstrating how nurses prepared in diploma, baccalaureate, and associate degree programs differ in their approaches to, and attitudes toward, nursing practice are far from conclusive. Research studies provide conflicting evidence about the effect the type of nursing education has on performance. The central issue facing nursing remains, "Are there two categories of nurses in practice and, if so, can the distinction between the two be made on the basis of education?" (Dennis & Janken, 1979, p. 37).

Studies attempting to delineate clearly the differences between technical and professional nursing found that each type of nurse performs most identified activities but in different proportions. Changes in health care are increasing the complexity of nursing. Nurses are required to provide more specialized services with increased use of technical equipment. There is more emphasis on recording details of care because of liability considerations. The need to differentiate between categories of nursing is becoming more necessary and more apparent.

It is equally important to provide feedback to educational programs as to the performance of graduates. Whereas nursing is attempting to classify categories and functions, education is attempting to decide which type of program best prepares the student for professional nursing practice.

Findings from Watson's (1982) study suggest that graduates of technical and professional programs are equally effective in identification skills. There are some possible explanations for these findings. The four components of the nursing process, of which problem identification is a part, are inherent in each type of educational program. Although, as the National League for Nursing (1979) points out, the extent of incorporation is different in "depth and breadth" of implementation. Associate degree programs have been lengthened beyond the original two-year concept (Montag, 1980). In some instances, it takes approximately as long to complete an associate degree program as it does to complete a baccalaureate degree program. The "extent" to which the nursing process is included in lengthened associate degree programs remains unclear.

In 1980, Montag commented that "there was an increasing tendency to teach associate degree students everything, with little discrimination as to what the technical nurse needs to know in order to deal with common recurring problems"

(p. 250). Kramer (1981) has also commented on the recent effort of associate degree programs to "become mini-baccalaureate programs" (p. 226). She contends, that, "in dedication to devotion to the cause of articulation, many ADN programs have tried to be or become all things to all people; they have included leadership, public health nursing content, and other content irrelevant to technical nursing...." (p. 226).

Service expectations may also be a contributing factor to the similarity in problem identification skills among graduates. All registered nurses, irrespective of type of educational preparation, are expected to assess, plan, implement, and evaluate patient care. All nurses are expected to develop and implement patient care plans. It is becoming increasingly crucial to differentiate functions according to type of educational preparation. Such differentiation is needed to guide program decisions and budgetary allocations in the educational setting.

As nursing continues to struggle for professional identity, the needs of nurses, the profession, and society must be incorporated. Choices must be made regarding which kind (type) of educational programs are needed to best meet these needs. The question of how many types of nurses are needed for optimal delivery of nursing services remains unanswered as does the question of whether or not there is a difference in the graduate's performance dependent upon educational route pursued.

Limitations of Research

The research to date is limited in generalizability due to methodological weaknesses. In the review of research dealing with cognitive development as a result of the professional socialization process, two recurring problems were noted: (1) small sample sizes, and (2) lack of control of extraneous variables. Some studies arrived at conclusions and interpretations based on a sample size limited to ten subjects. Other studies lacked equal representation, unequal samples, of programs being evaluated. Another problem frequently noted was that the reliability and validity of instruments used were not addressed.

Performance studies relied heavily on perceptions of others. It was noted that the ratings completed by supervisors may be biased due to their own educational preparation. In some studies, this variable was not identified nor controlled for.

Many studies suffered from a low response rate, 30-48%. Others suffered from poorly defined and tested instruments, and there were some which lacked statistical analysis. The limitations of the research reviewed support the need for additional research in the area of professional socialization of the registered nurse.

Implications For Future Research

Current evidence remains inadequate to tell whether graduates of different types of programs actually perform differently. Additional research is needed. Equally important is the need to determine if and how graduates are used differently in the service setting. The question is posed: if performance expectations in the service setting do not reflect differences in competencies, should education continue to struggle to produce different kinds of graduates.

Watson's (1982) study established an associative relationship between type of educational preparation and professional socialization of the registered nurse.

PROFESSIONAL SOCIALIZATION OF THE REGISTERED NURSE

According to her study, baccalaureate programs have produced nurses who have stronger attitudes of professionalism than nurse graduates of diploma and associate degree programs. Though the study did determine a relationship between type of educational preparation and effective problem identification skills, no significant difference in such skills was established for "technical" and "professional" performance.

The conclusions from this review of literature indicate the need for further study in the area of professional socialization of the registered nurse. Further studies should be undertaken to determine the relationship between the organizational environment and the manifestation of professional values. Additional testing of the problem solving abilities is recommended. The data from Watson's (1982) study suggests that generic baccalaureate graduates experience less reality shock than other graduates. Further testing is needed to validate these findings. And lastly, a longitudinal study is recommended to evaluate the socialization process throughout the educational process and into the work setting.

In conclusion, the determination of the effects of educational preparation on performance remains a relevant and timely issue for nursing. As a profession, nursing is responsible for educating nurses to meet current and emerging health care needs of society. In an effort to fulfill this professional responsibility, nursing has established baccalaureate education as the minimum preparation necessary for professional practice. Nursing has not, however, established differentiated functions according to type of educational preparation.

REFERENCES

Alutto, J.A., Hrebiniak, L.G., & Alonso, R.C. A study of differential socialization for members of one professional occupation. *Journal of Health and Social Behavior*, 1971, *12*, 140-147.

Bailey, J.T. New approaches to curriculum development. *Nursing Outlook*, 1966, *14*, 33-35.

Beverly, L., & Junker, M.H. The AD nurse: Prepared to be prepared. *Nursing Outlook*, 1977, *25*, 514-518.

Brown, J.S., Swift, Y.B., & Oberman, M.L. Baccalaureate students' images of nursing: A replication. *Nursing Research*, 1974, *23*, 53-59.

Bullough, B., & Sparks, C. Baccalaureate vs associate degree nurses: The care-cure dichotomy. *Nursing Outlook*, 1975, *23*, 688-692.

Chamings, P.A., & Treevan, J. Comparison of expected competencies of baccalaureate and associate degree graduates in nursing. *Image*, 1979, *11*, 16-21.

Cicatiello, J.S.A. Expectations of the associate degree nurses. *Journal of Nursing Education*, 1974, *13*(2), 22-25.

Cohen, H.A. *The nurse's quest for a professional identity*. Menlo Park, Calif: Addison-Wesley, 1981.

Corwin, R.G., Taves, M., & Haas, J. Professional disillusionment. *Nursing Research*, 1961, *10*, 141-144.

Davis, B.G. Clinical expertise as a function of educational preparation. *Nursing Research,* 1972, *21,* 530-534.

Davis, B.G. Effects of levels of nursing education on patient care. *Nursing Research,* 1974, *23,* 150-155.

Davis, C.K. Anticipatory socialization: Its effect on role conceptions, role deprivations, and adaptive role strategies of graduating student nurses in selected associate degree and baccalaureate degree programs (Doctoral dissertation, Syracuse University, 1972). *Dissertation Abstracts International,* 1973, *33,* 4358-B.

Davis, F., & Oleson, V.L. Baccalaureate students' images of nursing. *Nursing Research,* 1964, *13,* 8-15.

Davis, F., & Oleson, V.L. The career outlook of professionally educated women. *Psychiatry,* 1965, *28,* 334-345.

Dennis, L.C., & Janken, J.K. *The relationship between nursing education and performance: A critical review* (DHEW Pub. No. HRA 79-38). Hyattsville, Maryland: USDHEW, Division of Nursing, 1979.

Dustan, L.C. Characteristics of students in three types of nursing education programs. *Nursing Research,* 1964, *13,* 159-166.

Dyer, E.D., Cope, M.J., Monson, M.A., & Van Drimmelsen, J.B. Can job performance be predicted from biographical, personality, and administrative climate inventories? *Nursing Research,* 1972, *21,* 294-304.

Ehrat, K.S. Educational/career mobility: Antecedent of change. *Nursing and Health Care,* 1981, *11,* 487-527.

Eller, V.M. Role orientation toward professional nursing of students completing associate degree, diploma, and baccalaureate nursing educational programs (Doctoral dissertation, North Carolina State University at Raleigh, 1976). *Dissertation Abstracts International,* 1976, *37,* 2770-B.

Fogarty, B.E. Employment activity of baccalaureate and diploma nurses. *Research in Nursing and Health Care,* 1980, *3,* 95-100.

Fromm, L. The problem in nursing: Nurses! *Supervisor Nurse,* 1977, *8*(10), 15-16.

Goff, J.H. The image of nursing and job satisfaction of United States Air Force nurses (Doctoral dissertation, North Texas State University, 1973). *Dissertation Abstracts International,* 1973, *34,* 1607-B.

Gray, J.E., Murray, B.L.S., & Sawyer, J.R. Do graduates of technical and professional nursing programs differ in practice? *Nursing Research,* 1977, *26,* 368-373.

Haussman, R.K., Hegyvary, I.T., & Newman, J.F., Jr. *Monitoring quality of nursing care: Part II - Assessment and study of correlates.* Washington: U. S. Department of Health, Education, and Welfare, 1976.

Highrighter, M.E. Nurse characteristics and patient progress. *Nursing Research,* 1969, *18,* 484-501.

Hittleman, D.R. A model for a competency based teacher preparation program. *Teacher education forum 4*, 1976, 1-114 (ERIC Document Reproduction Service No. ED 128 307).

Hogsdell, M.O. Associate degree and baccalaureate graduates: Do they function differently? *American Journal of Nursing*, 1977, *77*, 1598-1600.

Hover, J. Diploma vs. degree nurses: Are they alike? *Nursing Outlook*, 1975, *23*, 684, 687.

Howell, F.J. Employers' evaluation of new graduates. *Nursing Outlook*, 1978, *26*, 448-451.

Hurka, S.J. The registered nurse as a professional employee: A study of perceived role orientations (Doctoral dissertation, University of Washington, 1971). *Dissertation Abstracts International*, 1971, *31*, 3655-A.

Jacobs, A.M. Clinical competencies of baccalaureate, A.D., and diploma nurses — Are they different? *Issues*, 1980, *1*(4), 1-3, 6.

Jacobs, A.M., Febers, G., Edwards, D.S., & Fitzpatrick, R. *Critical requirements for safe/effective nursing practice*. Kansas City, Mo.: American Nurses' Association, 1978.

Jacox, A. Professional socialization of nurses. *Journal of the New York State Nurses' Association*, 1973, *4*(4), 6-15.

Johnson, D.E. Competence in practice: Technical and professional. *Nursing Outlook*, 1966, *14*, 30-33.

Knox, J.E. The formation of nurse role conceptions: A study of baccalaureate nursing students (Doctoral dissertation, Columbia University, 1971). *Dissertation Abstracts International*, 1971, *32*, 1296-A.

Kramer, M. Philosophical foundations of baccalaureate nursing education. *Nursing Outlook*, 1981, *29*, 224-228.

Kramer, M. *Reality shock: Why nurses leave nursing*. St. Louis: C.V. Mosby, 1974.

Kramer, M., & Baker, C. The exodus: Can we prevent it? *Journal of Nursing Administration*, 1971, *1*, 15-30.

Kramer, M., & Schmalenberg, C.E. Bicultural training and new graduate role transformation. *Nursing Digest*, 1978, *5*(4), 1-7.

Kubat, J. Correlates of professional obsolescence. Part I. *Journal of Continuing Education*, 1975, *6*, 22-29.

Kubat, J. Correlates of professional obsolescence. Part II. *Journal of Continuing Education*, 1976, *7*, 18-22.

Mandrillo, M.P. A comparative study of the cognitive skills of the graduating baccalaureate degree and associate degree nursing students (Doctoral dissertation, Columbia University, 1969). *Dissertation Abstracts International*, 1970, *30*, 4222-B.

Mantheny, R. Technical nursing practice. In Department of Baccalaureate and Higher Degree Programs, *Shifting scene — Directions for practice*. New York: National League for Nursing, 1967.

May, W.T., & Ilardi, R.L. Image and stability of values of collegiate nursing students. *Nursing Research*, 1970, *19*, 359-361.

PROFESSIONAL SOCIALIZATION OF THE REGISTERED NURSE

McClosky, J.C. The effects of nursing education on job effectiveness: An overview of the literature. *Research in Nursing and Health,* 1981, *4,* 355-373.

Meleis, A.I., & Farrel, K.M. Operation concern: A study of senior nursing students in three nursing programs. *Nursing Research,* 1974, *23,* 461-468.

Montag, M. Looking back: Associate degree education in perspective. *Nursing Outlook,* 1980, *28,* 248-250.

Moore, M.A. A study of the extent to which specific behavioral objectives differentiate baccalaureate, diploma, and associate arts nursing education programs (Doctoral dissertation, University of Iowa, 1966). *Dissertation Abstracts International,* 1967, *27,* 3259-B.

National League for Nursing. NLN's task force cites differences in competencies and practice roles. *NLN News,* 1979, *27*(6), 1-3.

National League for Nursing. *Position statement on nursing roles — Scope and preparation* (Pub. No. 11-1893). New York: National League for Nursing, 1982.

Nelson, L.F. Competencies of nursing graduates in technical, communicative, and administrative skills. *Nursing Research,* 1978, *27,* 121-125.

Oleson, V.L., & Davis, F. Baccalaureate students' images of nursing: A follow-up report. *Nursing Research,* 1966, *15,* 151-158.

Petti, E.R. A study of the relationship between the three levels of nursing education and nurse competency as rated by patient and head nurse (Doctoral dissertation, Boston University, 1975). *Dissertation Abstracts International,* 1975, *35,* 7536-7537-A.

Polifroni, E.C. Problem solving ability of senior nursing students in preservice and inservice baccalaureate programs (Doctoral dissertation, Rutgers University, 1981). *Dissertation Abstracts International,* 1981, *42,* 1395-B.

Reichow, R.W., & Scott, R.E. Study compares graduates of two- three- and four-year programs. *Hospitals,* 1976, *50,* 95-100.

Rotkovitch, R. The AD nurse: A nursing service perspective. *Nursing Outlook,* 1976, *24,* 234-236.

Schlotfeldt, R.M. Educational requirements for registered nursing. In *Entry into registered nursing — Issues and problems* (Pub. No. 23-1685). New York: National League for Nursing, 1977.

Schwerian, P.M. Evaluating the performance of nurses: A multidimensional approach. *Nursing Research,* 1978, *27,* 347-351.

Schwerian, P.M. (Project Director). *Prediction of successful nursing performance.* (Part I and II, Pub. No. HRA 77-271). Washington: Department of Health, Education, and Welfare, 1977.

Schwerian, P.M. (Project Director). *Prediction of successful nursing performance* (Part III and IV, Pub. No. HRA 79-15). Washington: Department of Health, Education, and Welfare, 1979.

Scoloveno, M.A. Problem solving ability of senior nursing students in three program types (Doctoral dissertation, Rutgers University, 1981). *Dissertation Abstracts International,* 1981, 1396-B.

Sharp, W.H., & Anderson, J.C. Changes in nursing students' descriptions of the personality traits of the ideal nurse. *Measurement and Evaluation in Guidance,* 1972, *5,* 339-444.

Siegel, H. Professional socialization in two baccalaureate programs. *Nursing Research,* 1968, *17,* 403-407.

Simms, S. Nursing's dilemma — The battle for role determination. *Supervisor Nurse,* 1977, *8*(9), 29-31.

Smoyak, S.A. A panel study comparing self-reports of baccalaureate degree and diploma nurses before graduation and after their first work week experience in hospitals. In ANA's *Eighth Nursing Research Conference,* Albuquerque, N. Mex., March 15-17, 1972.

Stromberg, F.M. Relationship of sex role identity to occupational image of female nursing students. *Nursing Research,* 1976, *25,* 363-369.

Tetreault, A.I. Selected factors associated with professional attitudes of baccalaureate nursing students. *Nursing Research,* 1976, *25,* 49-53.

Thomas, J.C.T. Professional socialization of students in four types of nursing education programs (Doctoral dissertation, University of Florida, 1978). *Dissertation Abstracts International,* 1979, *39,* 5966-A.

Tschudin, M.S. Educational preparation needed by the nurse in the future. *Nursing Outlook,* 1964, *12,* 32-35.

Ventura, M. Related social behaviors of students in different types of nursing education programs. *International Journal of Nursing Studies,* 1976, *13,* 3-10.

Verhonick, P.J., Nichols, B.A., & McCarthy, R.T. I came, I saw, I responded: Nursing observation and action survey. *Nursing Research,* 1968, *17,* 38-44.

Wang, R., & Watson, J. The professional nurse: Roles, competencies, and characteristics. *Supervisor Nurse,* 1977, *8*(6), 69-71.

Waters, V.H., Chater, S.S., Vivier, M.L., Urrea, J.H., & Wilson, H.S. Technical and professional nursing: An explanatory study. *Nursing Research,* 1972, *21,* 124-131.

PROFESSIONAL SOCIALIZATION OF THE REGISTERED NURSE

Watson, A.B. Professional socialization of the registered nurse as measured by attitudes and problem identification skills (Doctoral dissertation, University of California, San Francisco, 1982). Submitted to Dissertation Abstracts International, 1982.

Watson, D.L. Professional and technical function in nursing (Doctoral dissertation, Columbia University, Teachers College, 1979). *Dissertation Abstracts International,* 1981, *42,* 571-B.

Watson, J. Role conflict in nursing. *Supervisor Nurse,* 1977, *8*(7), 50.

Welches, L.J., Dixon, F.A., & Stanford, E.D. Typological prediction of staff nurse performance rating. *Nursing Research,* 1974, *23,* 402-409.

Werner, M.A. Professional socialization of nurses: A faculty member's view. *Journal of the New York State Nurses' Association,* 1973, *4*(4), 23-25.

Zarett, A. Is the BSN better? *RN,* 1980, *43*(3), 28-33; 78.

Chapter Three:
Research on Clinical Teaching

Chapter Three:
Research on Clinical Teaching

Elizabeth J. Pugh, Ph.D., R.N.

INTRODUCTION

Studies of the clinical teaching of nursing have focused almost exclusively on the perceptions of students, and have been undertaken primarily in an effort to identify important teaching behaviors which could then be used for the evaluation of faculty (Grebremedhin, 1974; Heidgerken, 1952; Jacobson, 1966; Layton, 1969). Only recently have investigators (Brodkorb, 1979; Brown, 1981; O'Shea & Parsons, 1979; Pugh, 1980; Stafford, 1979) sought perceptions of both students and faculty regarding desirable behavior of the clinical teacher.

A few investigators have studied a particular aspect of the role of the clinical teacher (Infante, 1975; Karns & Schwab, 1982; Rauen, 1974) and one investigator (Mannion, 1968) tried to develop a taxonomy of clinical instructional behaviors. The process of clinical teaching, analyzed from the perspective of the teacher, has been reported by Pugh (1980).

This dearth of reported studies is surprising in view of the fact that clinical experiences are considered to be an integral and necessary component of professional education. The major portion of a nursing student's learning experience, comprising 12 to 20 (or more) clock hours each week, is spent in the clinical setting. Although classroom teaching of nursing can be evaluated using tools of other disciplines in higher education, there are no accepted, established criteria for the evaluation of the clinical teaching of nursing. Indeed, there seems to be no commonly accepted, described, or communicated methodology of effective clinical teaching in any discipline.

Review of the Literature

The earliest reported study of nursing faculty was done by Loretta Heidgerken in 1952. Senior students (*n* = 384) in 37 schools of nursing (7 collegiate and 30 hospital programs) located in 21 states evaluated all the teachers they had had during their nursing school experience. Nursing students were asked to select their best and poorest teacher, and to describe the personal qualities and teaching activities. The inclusion of all types of faculty — physicians, college professors, dieticians, and occupational therapists as well as nursing faculty — contaminated the findings. The qualities and behaviors described by the sample were primarily applicable to classroom teaching; most related to skills required for lecture or class discussion. One quality stressed by the nursing students was "good example." Heidgerken believed that this behavior pertained to teaching in clinical settings, where the student would have had the opportunity to "observe the teaching in the actual practice of nursing, through demonstrations, ward conferences and clinics, as well as when she is teaching them" in classroom settings (Heidgerken, 1952, pp. 88).

Since Heidgerken's pioneering attempt to establish criteria for evaluation of nursing faculty, nursing students have been surveyed and interviewed in numerous efforts to determine effective classroom teaching behavior (Armington, Reinikka &

Creighton, 1972; Barham, 1965; Butler & Geitgey, 1970; Dixon & Koerner, 1976; Guthrie, 1953; Hassenplug, 1965; Jackson, 1977; Jacobson, 1966; Kiker, 1973; Lowery, Keane & Hyman, 1971; Mims, 1970; Wood, 1971a, 1971b). In spite of the use of different populations (students from diploma, associate degree, and baccalaureate programs), the lists of perceived effective classroom teaching behaviors have been strikingly similar. All of the studies of classroom teaching reported student and/or faculty beliefs about what constitutes effective teaching; observational descriptions of the behavior of effective classroom teachers cannot be found.

Studies of clinical teaching (Brodkorb, 1979; Brown, 1981; Grebremedhin, 1974; Infante, 1975; Jacobson, 1966; Karns & Schwab, 1982; Layton, 1969; Mannion, 1968; O'Shea & Parsons, 1979; Pugh, 1980; Rauen, 1973; Stafford, 1979) have also reported student and/or faculty beliefs about effective teacher behaviors. To facilitate review of these studies, they are grouped according to their type and source of data: Opinions of Students, Opinions of Students and Faculty, and Investigations Analyzing the Process of Clinical Teaching.

OPINIONS OF STUDENTS   Jacobson (1966) studied effective and ineffective nursing teacher behavior as defined by nursing students (n = 961) in five Southern university schools of nursing. Using a modified form of the critical incident technique (Flanagan, 1954) students generated 1,182 usable critical incidents during group interviews. Fifty-eight critical requirements for the teaching of nursing — both classroom and clinical — were derived and placed into six major categories. The categories were: availability of students, apparent knowledge and professional competence, interpersonal relationships with students and others, teaching practices in classroom and clinical areas, personal characteristics, and evaluation practices.

Although based entirely on the student perspective, and dealing with both clinical and classroom teaching, the representation of both public and private schools distributed throughout the South and the method of data collection made this study worthy of attention. Nearly every study of clinical teaching which followed its publication has in some way used the list of critical requirements identified by Jacobson.

Layton (1969) surveyed students (n = 141) in one diploma program in Detroit to determine which attitudes and actions of clinical instructors the students found helpful and which hindered their learning. Two open-ended questions were used. The most helpful attitudes and actions cited were those that demonstrated acceptance of the student as a person. Those hindering learning most often included a threatening or sarcastic approach, too close supervision, and being corrected in the presence of others. The investigator noted that these attitudes and actions were more closely related to the human relationships between faculty and students than to the content being taught.

A study by Rauen (1974) was designed to ascertain if diploma nursing students (n = 84) in three diploma programs in Milwaukee expected their clinical instructor to be a role model, defined as an effective nurse, measured by nurse role characteristics. An investigator-constructed rating scale was used which contained items describing behaviors which were descriptive of the teacher as Nurse, Teacher, and Person, based on the assumption that the clinical instructor portrayed those major roles to the student.

The subjects ranked Nurse role characteristics as significantly more important than Person or Teacher role characteristics in helping them become the type of nurses they wished to become. Three out of four of the priority instructor characteristics were Nurse role characteristics: "Demonstrate how to function in a real nursing situation," "Shows a contagious enthusiasm for giving quality patient care," "Shows a continued interest in applying improved methods of giving nursing care," and "Encourages me to think for myself." Freshman students ranked the clinical instructor's role characteristics as significantly more important than either Person role or Teacher role characteristics. Seniors ranked the Nurse role and Person role characteristics as equally important in helping them to learn to be nurses.

In an effort to pursue the findings of Rauen and Layton, as well as those of Barham (1965) and Jacobson (1966), Grebremedhin (1974) sought to identify those instructor qualities perceived by sophomore and senior nursing students as most helpful in facilitating their clinical nursing experience. She wanted to determine if baccalaureate students discriminated between affective and cognitive qualities of teachers.

Affective qualities of teachers were defined as teacher behaviors which involve interaction with the individual student, "for the purpose of providing insight into the students' feelings" (Grebremedhin, 1974, p. 11). Cognitive qualities were defined as "teacher behaviors which involve or facilitate thinking, knowing, or development of intellectual abilities" on the part of the learner (Grebremedhin, 1974, p. 12).

An investigator-constructed instrument, consisting of 20 teacher qualities derived from both nursing and non-nursing studies, was administered to sophomores (n = 27) and seniors (n = 27) in one Northwestern baccalaureate program. The items selected most frequently by the total sample — "Shows respect for your questions and opinions," "Increases your skill in thinking," "Demonstrates interest in and acceptance of you as a person," "Shows genuine interest in patients and their care," and "Uses class time efficiently" — reflect both affective and cognitive qualities. No significant differences were found between the sophomore and senior students.

Karns and Schwab (1982) asked 31 junior baccalaureate students in one program to list five teacher behaviors which they felt promoted a positive relationship between faculty and students. All students listed behaviors which could be categorized in at least two, and several in three interpersonal techniques emphasized by Aspy (1972): empathy, congruence (honesty), and positive regard (respect). The investigators related that Aspy's extensive research on use of interpersonal skills has shown that use of these skills in public school teaching can reduce student stress as well as relate to higher achievement, cognitive growth, and increased levels of critical thinking in students. They encouraged faculty to evaluate their own use of empathy, congruence, and positive regard in their interactions with their own students.

OPINIONS OF STUDENTS AND FACULTY More recent studies of beliefs about effective clinical teaching have sought data from both students and faculty.

This trend in design allows for comparisons to be made between faculty and student responses to similar items.

Brodkorb (1979) surveyed both faculty ($n = 125$) and students ($n = 1,130$) in nine schools of nursing in Illinois, representing diploma, associate degree, and baccalaureate nursing programs. The purpose of her master's thesis was to identify the relative importance of selected instructor behaviors and to determine if there were behaviors universally identified by students and faculty in all three types of programs.

Using an investigator-developed instrument containing 34 behavioral items, faculty and students rated the importance of each behavior, and then selected the five most important and the five least important behaviors. Questionnaires were stratified according to type of program, school, and status of respondent (faculty or student), and one-third of the questionnaires were randomly chosen for analysis within each strata.

Faculty and students in all programs selected the same two behaviors as the most important: "Allows me to function as independently as I am able" and "Relates with honest, forthright manner my specific strengths and weaknesses." Although no significant differences were found between overall faculty and student responses, it was reported that important faculty behaviors vary among the three types of educational programs, e.g., the behavior pertaining to honest evaluation was significantly more important to students in baccalaureate programs, and students in diploma programs were significantly more indifferent to the behavior, "Serves as a role model."

O'Shea and Parsons' (1979) sample consisted of 205 students and 24 faculty in the baccalaureate nursing program of one private Southern university. Students were requested to list on one side of a card three to five teacher behaviors that facilitated their learning in the clinical setting; three to five behaviors that interfered with their learning were to be listed on the other side of the card. The faculty were asked to complete identical cards, listing behaviors they believed facilitated or hindered student learning.

Responses were sorted into three broad categories designated as Evaluative behaviors, Instructive/Assistive behaviors, and Personal characteristics. Evaluative behaviors consisted of those which described feedback from teacher to student relative to the student's clinical performance or written work. Instructive/Assistive behaviors were viewed as those which supported the student in performing motor skills required for clinical nursing and intellectual processes essential for application of the nursing process. Assistive behaviors required the teacher to become physically involved with the task; instructive behaviors occurred more often during verbal exchange. Personal characteristics developed either the personality of the teacher or the teaching practices which were not easily identified with the other two categories.

Data were analyzed according to the level of student (junior, senior) and faculty status, and were presented according to the three categories of behaviors. Agreement was found between students and faculty regarding the importance of the use of feedback to facilitate student learning. Faculty availability was the behavior noted by all groups to be the most important within the Instructive/Assistive category. The most marked difference found between faculty and students was in regard to role modeling: faculty indicated role modeling as a facilitative behavior five times more often than students did. The investigators suggested that the faculty member's definition of role modeling may be broader than that of students, who may define role modeling primarily as a demonstration of nursing procedures.

To determine the behaviors and characteristics of effective clinical teaching in nursing, Stafford (1979) developed a 60-item instrument through a Delphi process. This elicited input from nursing educators, practicing graduates, and senior nursing students in the state of Texas. The samples were obtained through an elaborate multilevel nomination process. Four of the seven state-supported baccalaureate programs in the State of Texas agreed to participate. The sample consisted of 95 faculty and 189 senior students, obtained through an unreported process, and 120 Texas nurses with baccalaureate degrees, randomly selected from a list obtained from the State Board of Examiners. When respondents were asked to rate the importance of each item, the three groups of subjects agreed that behaviors such as functioning as a role model for students, identifying important clinical content, and providing opportunities for students to practice problem solving and technical skills were very important. Students placed high value on being treated as colleagues by faculty, but educators viewed this behavior as less important.

Pugh (1980) surveyed beliefs of the importance of 20 observable clinical teaching behaviors from 50 randomly selected faculty and their students ($n = 358$) from eight randomly selected baccalaureate programs in the state of Illinois. All levels and types of students were represented; faculty represented all clinical specialties. Faculty and their respective students completed questionnaires administered by the investigator during a conference in their clinical setting.

Both faculty and students rated the importance of 20 clinical teaching behaviors on a 7-point scale, from "minor" to "essential." The questionnaire was constructed from an initial list of 27 behaviors reported to be helpful in previous studies (Jacobson, 1966; Mannion, 1968). Items were subjected to review by a group of experienced nurse faculty experts ($n = 17$), selected to represent undergraduate master's-prepared faculty.

To explore the structure of the ratings, the students' ratings of the importance of the behaviors were subjected to an exploratory factor analysis with varimax rotation. Five factors were identified: Teacher, Nurse, Evaluation, Application, Guidance. Students in the sample expected their clinical faculty member to be primarily a Teacher, enacting teaching behaviors directed at the student as a learner, and secondly, a Nurse, enacting behaviors which included helping students put together data about their patients, interacting with students' patients/families, encouragement of professionalism, and demonstration of how to function in a real nursing situation. Six of the eight behaviors rated highest by students in this sample loaded on Factor 1, Teacher, with the most highly-rated behavior being, "Demonstrate how to function in a real nursing situation."

Faculty agreed that all 20 teaching behaviors were important; the five most highly rated were in order: showing interest in students, commenting on written assignments, encouraging student self-evaluation, giving positive reinforcement, and serving as a resource person. Although faculty and students agreed on the relative importance of only one behavior appearing in their lists of those most highly rated ("Correct and comment on written assignments"), both lists contained items which indicated a degree of agreement regarding the use of feedback in clinical teaching.

Among the 20 importance ratings by students, there were only six instructional behaviors which differed significantly among different types and levels of students. R.N. students consistently ascribed less importance to the clinical instructor's demonstrating how to function as a nurse, observing while they are engaged in patient care, and giving them opportunity to practice before evaluation. Seniors rated help with synthesis of patient data and contact with their patients as significantly less important than juniors rated these items. Seniors rated observation of their patient care significantly lower than either sophomores or juniors.

The clinical setting also had an effect upon student importance ratings. Students in public health nursing gave significantly lower ratings than students in obstetrics for the importance of the teacher demonstrating how to function as a nurse and observing them while giving care. Public health nursing students also ascribed significantly more importance to the encouragement of self-evaluation than students in pediatric settings. Students in obstetrics gave significantly higher ratings than did students in psychiatric settings for the teacher's interaction with their patients and families.

A national survey of faculty in nursing, medicine, and dentistry was done with the intent to gather and assess information useful in the "designation and implementation of clinical teaching improvement programs in the health sciences" (Meleca, Schimpfhauser, Witteman, & Sachs, 1981). Items of clinical teaching behavior for each discipline were obtained through observation of experienced faculty by trained raters and submission of critical incidents by students.

The survey of nursing faculty included 672 faculty in all types of nursing programs (n = 119). In addition to providing demographic and professional data, each respondent indicated the type of teaching that best typified his/her clinical teaching. As would be expected, clinical supervision (72%), small group seminars (16%), one-to-one conferences with students (8%), and lecturing to student (4%) were reported as the type of encounters most often utilized. Subjects were also asked to indicate their actual and ideal use of each teaching skill. Skills were categorized as (a) presentation, (b) questioning, (c) attending, and (d) teaching styles. Teaching categories of presentation, i.e., "Informing students of objectives of upcoming learning experiences," and questioning were reported to be utilized more than the perceived ideal, while attending, i.e., "Answer students' questions during a teaching session," and behaviors in the category of teaching styles, i.e., "Assist students in undertaking issues which affect the profession of nursing" were reported to be used less than the faculty members' perceived ideal.

The heavy reliance upon self-reported data, the mix of faculty from all types of nursing programs, the lack of distinction between types of programs, and the incompleteness of the article (which was apparently intended to inform nurse educators) render the findings of little importance or assistance in the description or analysis of the clinical teaching of nursing.

Brown (1981) surveyed senior nursing students (n = 82) and faculty (n = 42) in one Southern university in order to determine how baccalaureate students and faculty compare in their description of characteristics of effective clinical teachers.

Using an investigator-constructed instrument, subjects rated the relative importance of 20 teacher characteristics (a combination of instruction behaviors and personal attributes), and then selected and ranked the five characteristics they believed were most important. The students regarded the instructor's relationships with students as more important than professional competence, while faculty regarded items describing professional competence as more important than those describing teacher-student relationships. Both groups ranked two items as among the five most important: "Provides useful feedback on student progress," and "Is objective and fair in the evaluation of the student."

The studies described so far assessed perceptions of students and/or faculty about effective teaching behaviors. Only three studies exist in which the process is analyzed from the perspective of the teacher.

INVESTIGATIONS ANALYZING THE PROCESS OF CLINICAL
TEACHING Infante (1975) studied the extent to which clinical laboratory activities in selected baccalaureate programs in nursing characterized the essential elements of the laboratory concept. Her study was based upon an unpublished dissertation (Zasowska, 1967) which examined the laboratory experience and in which the investigator had concluded that the clinical laboratory in nursing was obscurely defined and ambiguously identified. Infante believed that emphasis should not be on how to care for patients, but on how to apply knowledge to the care of patients (Infante, 1975, p. 23).

A self-administered, mailed questionnaire constructed by the investigator was used to determine the beliefs and reported current practices engaged in by faculty in selected baccalaureate programs in New England. In addition to personal data, the questionnaire contained items the respondents believed laboratory activities should include, or what they said they did in the clinical laboratory. The final section included a description of situations in clinical teaching. Respondents were asked to select one of three options which described the way they would handle the situation. Options were written for each situation to reflect sound educational practice which would be employed if the teacher were properly utilizing the laboratory concept; the worker-oriented approach to teaching in the clinical laboratory, where the emphasis was on task performance, not student learning; and a mixture of activities which represented some aspects of the laboratory concept and some aspects of worker-oriented approach to teaching (Infante, 1975, p. 67).

The investigator found that the laboratory concept — which essentially defined the student as learner, not as responsible care giver — was utilized by a low to moderate percentage of nursing faculty. She reported a striking contrast between what the faculty stated they believed and what they practiced. Many faculty expressed a belief in the laboratory concept, yet few gave evidence of practicing this concept. The determination of the reasons for that finding was not within the scope of the study. Infante admitted to a need for data collection by direct observation of faculty in order to verify that inconsistencies do indeed exist.

Two studies of clinical teaching (Mannion, 1968; Pugh, 1980) included direct observation of the clinical teaching of a sample of faculty. The purpose of Mannion's dissertation was to develop a taxonomy of instructional behaviors applicable to the guidance of learning activities in the clinical setting in baccalaureate nursing education; her observation of faculty was done for the purpose of validating that taxonomy.

Mannion first located 30 investigations in nursing and related fields which have clinical or field instruction as an integral part of the curriculum. Extracting instructional behaviors, she placed them into a meaningful organizational framework. Modification of the classification was made on the basis of input from a jury of experts.

A small observational study in one Southwestern baccalaureate program assisted the investigator to determine the applicability of the classification in the clinical setting and to develop sensitivity for placing overt behaviors in her categories. The investigator accompanied five faculty for three separate half-hour periods during one clinical teaching day. Observations were not recorded during the course of the observations. The investigator withdrew from the setting and reconstructed the situation, then checked the overt behaviors which were observed during the time period on a schedule which listed all behaviors on the taxonomy. A total of 310 instructional behaviors were observed during 15 half-hour periods. Some changes were made in the original statement of behaviors in the taxonomy, and one new behavior was added.

The final phase consisted of collecting instructional behaviors which described instructor-student interactions in the clinical setting. Using an adapted critical incident technique, 226 descriptions of instructional interactions with undergraduate students were obtained from 52 volunteer faculty from six baccalaureate programs in one state. A total of 1,560 instructional behaviors were tabulated and presented in numerical and descriptive form, forming a taxonomy (Mannion, 1968, pp. 64-68).

Mannion (1968) concluded that the process of clinical instruction consisted of behaviors which were classified as (a) information-gathering about the student and the clinical setting in which the student acquired practice experience; (b) assessment and interpretation, which involved a direct encounter between the instructor and the student in the clinical setting; and (c) instrumental, which implied active intervention on the part of the instructor in the clinical instructional process (p. 96).

With one exception (Pugh, 1980), the investigations of clinical teaching which followed Mannion's dissertation (Brodkorb, 1969; Brown, 1981; Grebremedhin, 1974; Infante, 1975; Karns & Schwab, 1982; Layton, 1969; Meleca, et al., 1981; O'Shea & Parsons, 1979; Rauen, 1974; Stafford, 1979) gave no indication of having reviewed it. It is possible that because Mannion's findings were not reported outside *Dissertation Abstracts*, the study has remained virtually unknown to investigators studying clinical teaching.

Troubled by the paucity and simplicity of research on clinical teaching, and intrigued by Infante's findings, Pugh (1980) explored factors affecting the apparent discrepancy between what nursing faculty state they believe to be important teaching behaviors and those they actually implement. Fishbein-Ajzen's theory of reasoned action (Ajzen & Fishbein, 1980; Fishbein & Ajzen, 1975) was combined with significant aspects of role enactment — role expectations, role preparation, role skills, referent groups — in an effort to explain and predict teacher behavior. Twenty clinical teaching behaviors based upon the Fishbein-Ajzen model were rated on the following scales: evaluation of the importance; the probability of use; perception of the probability with which their fellow faculty would expect them to use the behavior; the probability with which their students would expect them to use the behavior; attitude toward the behavior; and rating of the behavior as they perceive their fellow faculty would rate it.

Part II of the Faculty Questionnaire consisted of two identical 16-scale semantic differentials — "Myself as a Teacher," "Myself as a Nurse" — which elucidated perceptions of social roles as teacher and as nurse. In Part III, Professional and Educational Data, faculty indicated how they described themselves, i.e., "I am a nurse," "I am a teacher," "I am a nurse who teaches nursing," etc.

The Student Questionnaire consisted of the same twenty teaching behaviors. All items were considered to be of low inference and directly observable by students. Students were also asked to rate the importance of each behavior on a 7-point scale, from 1, "minor" to 7, "essential." On a second 7-point scale they were to indicate the frequency with which their clinical instructor used each behavior, from 1, "never" to 7, "very often."

Fifty faculty were observed by the investigator for one entire clinical day teaching in a patient care setting. Observations were used in order to verify students' reports, to document and describe patterns of behavior, and to provide an opportunity to study the contextual background of teacher behavior. This sample of nursing faculty reported that they believed in the importance of the 20 teaching behaviors, had generally positive attitudes toward them, and perceived their faculty peers as expecting them to use the behaviors. However, their behavior did not follow directly from their stated intentions to use each behavior, i.e., students did not indicate they engaged in the behaviors.

Reasons for lack of apparent congruence between intention and behavior were hypothesized by the investigator. These included problems in measurement of complex, multifaceted behavior; students' definitions of some behaviors, e.g., role modeling, which did not coincide with those held by faculty; and lack of opportunity for faculty to perform the intended behavior. Using role theory to explain incongruence, ignorance of role expectations, inability to perform as a result of inadequate preparation, and absence of motivation to meet the role expectations were cited as possible reasons for non-performance.

The majority of faculty in this sample identified themselves as nurses who teach nursing. Neither role identification nor role preparation alone had a significant effect on behavioral intentions, attitude toward specific behaviors, or perceived attitude of faculty peers. There were very few behaviors which showed differences in ratings of importance, faculty perceptions of students' expectations, and peer expectations when analyzed according to role identification or role preparation.

Three distinct patterns of faculty behavior were observed: Nurse, Teacher, and Nurse-Teacher. Nurses enacted primarily nurse behaviors; Teachers enacted teacher behaviors; and Nurse-Teachers appeared comfortable using behaviors appropriate to both roles. Faculty role identification did not in itself predict the observed behavior of faculty. However, when role identification was combined with role preparation and value placed on teaching or clinical practice, congruence between the three variables predicted observed behavior.

Synthesis

Research in clinical teaching of nursing is in its infancy. Most of the studies are exploratory and descriptive in nature, report students' perceptions of importance of a variety of teacher characteristics or behaviors, and use primarily univariate analyses. Few investigators have utilized adequate theory to explain clinical teaching.

It is difficult to compare findings across surveys when different instruments and methodologies are used. Study methodologies have primarily consisted of: (a) a generation of items by students or faculty, (b) a ranking of a given set of items, or (c) a rating of the importance of observable teaching behaviors and/or personal characteristics of the teacher. For these reasons, it does not seem fruitful to construct a table which would integrate all of the teacher behaviors reported to be important to student learning in the clinical setting.

In spite of these methodological and measurement problems, there is some consensus of opinion about three categories of desirable teacher behavior with undergraduate students in the clinical setting: (a) teacher-student relationships, (b) use of feedback, and (c) enactment of both teacher and nurse roles by nurse faculty. Each category is summarized.

TEACHER-STUDENT RELATIONSHIPS Behaviors or characteristics of faculty which demonstrate positive regard for the student were reflected in the findings of several investigators. Showing respect for students' questions and opinions (Grebremedhin, 1974; Karns & Schwab, 1982); being treated as a colleague (Stafford, 1979); and showing confidence in and respect for the student and having realistic expectations for students (Brown, 1981; Karns & Schwab, 1982) were rated or ranked among the most important teacher behaviors. Brown concluded that her sample of baccalaureate students regarded the instructor's relationship with students as more important than professional competence, a notion which is lent support by Karn's & Schwab's students, who listed personal characteristics of empathy, honesty, and respect as the most facilitative behaviors or characteristics of faculty.

Both diploma (Layton, 1969) and baccalaureate (Grebremedhin, 1974; Karns & Schwab, 1982; Pugh, 1980) students revealed that it was important for the faculty member to demonstrate interest in and acceptance of the student as a person. When given the opportunity to add items, 34 of the 67 behaviors added by undergraduates in Pugh's sample described interactional aspects of teacher-learner relationship: "Don't talk down to students," "Realize that students are human," "Support students after mistakes," "Recognize when I am not myself and ask if I want to talk." This finding led the investigator to wonder about the degree of empathy conveyed by faculty in interactions with students.

USE OF FEEDBACK In studies examining both students' and faculty's perceptions of helpful teaching behaviors, both groups agreed on the importance of the use of feedback. Desirable evaluation is described as objective and fair (Brown, 1981); and should be related to the student in private (Layton, 1969); in an honest, forthright and positive manner (Brodkorb, 1979; Karns & Schwab, 1982). Constructive criticism should be provided (Brown, 1979; O'Shea & Parsons, 1979), and specific suggestions should be given for improvement (Pugh, 1980).

ENACTMENT OF TEACHER AND NURSE ROLES Two investigators have specifically studied the role of nursing faculty. Rauen's (1974) study of diploma students suggested that these students believed that the faculty member's role as Nurse was significantly more important than her roles of Teacher or Person. Baccalaureate students (Pugh, 1980) clearly indicated that they expected their faculty to enact both Teacher and Nurse roles.

Opinion studies of clinical teaching have provided data which indicate that faculty are expected to be both a role model as a nurse and to enact specific instructional behaviors which are enacted by teachers, i.e., provide feedback, help students apply theory to clinical situations, evaluate fairly, etc. It seems reasonable that faculty who teach students in a practice profession must be concerned not only with the role modeling they do as nurses, but also with their role as a teacher who manipulates the clinical environment to provide learning experiences for students (Infante, 1975).

Implications

Knowledge of students' perceptions about which clinical teaching behaviors are helpful to them has implications for both nursing education and faculty development. Faculty can be encouraged to utilize behavior which is reported to be helpful, i.e., provision of feedback immediately following an observed situation, returning written work with helpful comments and directions for future improvement, verbal feedback as often as possible. Faculty who were prepared as clinicians — not as teachers of clinical nursing — can learn those instructional skills desired by students.

Data from several of the studies reviewed in this chapter (Brown, 1981; Grebremedhin, 1974; Karns & Schwab, 1982; Layton, 1969; Pugh, 1980) revealed that students want to be accepted, listened to, and treated with respect. While clinical teaching behaviors are able to be learned, development of interpersonal skills facilitative of students' learning is perhaps a different matter, and more closely related to a teacher's philosophy of teaching-learning (Brunclik, Thurston & Feldhusen, 1967; Karns & Schwab, 1982; Pugh, 1976).

A faculty member whose clinical teaching requires enactment of two professional roles — teacher and practitioner — needs time and opportunity to maintain and improve competence in both roles. This notion implies support for institutions which provide for faculty to be employed in joint education and practice positions; students can observe faculty legitimately enacting both teacher and practitioner roles.

One must be careful, however, that the teacher's enactment of the practitioner role is intentional, e.g., enacted for the purpose of providing the student with a learning experience which assists in the application of theory to clinical patient situations. It has been demonstrated (O'Shea & Parsons, 1979; Pugh, 1980) that undergraduate students cannot be depended upon to identify when a faculty member is "being a role model," therefore, any teacher's demonstration of nurse behaviors should be carefully planned, explained and evaluated. To simply behave as a nurse in the presence of a student may not produce the desired student behavior in a similar situation at some future time.

Insight into the determinants of faculty behavior provides directions for graduate programs in nursing. Preparation at the graduate level usually provides for development of specialized role skills and anticipatory socialization to one role. Expectations of dual role enactment in undergraduate professional education requires that nursing faculty achieve complementarity between two roles which are inherently quite separate with different, and often conflicting, role expectations.

Many graduates of programs which prepare clinical specialists will eventually take faculty positions for which they will be unprepared. Efforts must be made to expose graduate students to the educational aspects of the practitioner role, e.g., knowledge about learning theory, instructional design, and evaluation, which will be encountered in their roles as clinical specialists and providers of continuing education. Core courses which encompass educational theory used by nurses practicing in a variety of settings should be part of every graduate program in nursing (McKay, 1971). This basic theory could later be expanded by well-organized and effective faculty development programs, where application could be made to the teaching of young professionals.   A recent study to identify common core competencies of master's prepared nurses (McLane, 1978) also emphasized the importance of practitioner competencies for teachers. The future teacher should have opportunities to continue development of clinical skills beyond that obtained at the baccalaureate level, but the primary emphasis of such programs should be on the functional role of teacher.

Limitations

Although each of the studies reviewed has provided interesting data, a number of problems can be identified which limit the generalizability of findings. Limitations of the research currently available in the area of clinical teaching can be described according to the samples, methodology, and dissemination of findings.

SAMPLES   Sampling problems have plagued many studies: use of volunteers, generally small samples limited to one institution, and unclear methods of sampling greatly limit generalizability. It is almost as though each study was designed totally in isolation from the literature, unsupported by sufficient financial aid to allow for comparison groups or institutions, and without consultation from researchers skilled in sampling methodology. Very few investigators attempted to randomly sample either students or faculty from more than one institution.

METHODOLOGY   The primary method utilized, opinion survey, in itself limits usefulness. Dependence upon the students' perspective may be seen by some as a limitation. Others will consider such use as quite appropriate, for it is the learner who is the best reporter of what is helpful to him in such a situation (Costin, Greenough & Menges, 1971; Menges, 1979).

Although most investigators reported utilizing Jacobson's (1966) list of critical requirements in the construction of their own instrument, no two studies have used the same questionnaire. As a result, the findings of each study are relative to the questionnaire used; only those items listed are rated. Also, the studies are very difficult to compare. There is little evidence of continuation of efforts or building upon previous research in the area. Additionally, there is no evidence that any of the investigators have continued to research the same topical area or ever replicated their own (or someone else's) previous work. This is a serious limitation, causing each new researcher to again try to "reinvent the wheel."

Researchers have been interested only in the perception of undergraduate students; none have reported perceptions of graduate students. The two earliest studies utilized diploma students; later studies have surveyed only baccalaureate students. Only one investigator reported differences in ratings between generic baccalaureate students and those of registered nurse students.

Analyses have utilized mostly descriptive statistics, presenting means or ranks of items descriptive of faculty behavior or personality. Few attempts have been made to examine differences in student preferences other than by level of student or type of program. Only one investigator analyzed ratings among levels of students, type of student, number of previous clinical instructors, and type of clinical setting. These analytic deficits may be in part due to the limits imposed by small, non-random samples and the meager amount of demographic data obtained.

One investigator reported teachers' actual behavior and attempted to analyze factors affecting such behavior from the teacher perspective. Her use of observation to document and describe teaching behavior provided an objective description of behavior and events not possible through self-report. A recent review of research (Hook & Rosenshine, 1979) revealed that one cannot assume that teachers' reports of their classroom behavior will in any way be accurate; one should not expect that clinical faculty would be any more accurate. Use of more than one source of data, e.g., teacher's self-report, students as multiple raters, observer as rater, is one step in the direction of obtaining more than just student opinion or teacher self-report.

DISSEMINATION OF FINDINGS Although studies have been reported in local, regional or even national meetings, the findings have had limited exposure. Those which are available only through interlibrary loan (Brodkorb, 1979; Grebremedhin, 1974) or in *Dissertation Abstracts International* (Mannion, 1968; Pugh, 1980; Stafford, 1979) are not readily accessible to potential researchers. Some of the later dissertations may just now be finding their way into print as journal articles. Others (Karns & Schwab, 1982; Layton, 1969; O'Shea & Parsons, 1979) perhaps were limited by editorial policy and were unable to provide reports which were sufficiently detailed to allow replication.

Future Research

We have only begun to move beyond exploratory and descriptive research in clinical teaching. There are tentative descriptions of teaching behaviors which students cite, rate, or rank as important to their learning in the clinical setting. There is need to analyze the process of clinical teaching using appropriate theory to guide our efforts.

A variety of research methods should be utilized to examine a multidimensional activity such as clinical teaching. Students' viewpoints, as reported in the great majority of studies reviewed, are certainly one important source of data for identifying characteristics of effective clinical teachers. Faculty members' viewpoints, reported in fewer studies and studied less vigorously, are important in that they allow us to better understand the perceptual world of the person enacting the behavior. Use of behavioral observation to study clinical teaching provides advantages over the use of questionnaires alone. Observation provides an opportunity to study the contextual background of teacher behavior in a complex setting. It would not have been possible, for instance, for Pugh (1980) to have discovered that patterns of nursing faculty behavior existed if only self-report and student ratings had been utilized.

Effective clinical teaching may be the result of utilizing specific patterns of instruction which are based on the characteristics of the nursing student, the content to be applied in the clinical setting, or some combination of factors not yet identified. Regardless of the patterns of instruction, it does appear that the actions of the teacher are intentional: she plans to enact specific behaviors for the purpose of facilitating the students' learning. Validation of the effectiveness of the teacher behaviors which have been rated by students as helpful is a neglected area of research. Appropriate outcome measures of student performance need to be devised for validation of teacher behaviors.

Hawkins (1981) developed a model for the selection of clinical agencies which provide optimal clinical experiences for students. Her study was not reviewed here since it examined teacher behavior which, although related to planning for clinical experiences, does not directly involve teacher-student interaction in the clinical setting. However, such studies which examine faculty responsibilities that impact upon where clinical teaching occurs are also important to pursue.

One direction which requires study and which has implications for preparation of faculty is the exploration of the effectiveness of nursing faculty who differ in role identity. Is the Nurse-Teacher the best model? The ability to enact both roles fit the "importance" ratings of baccalaureate students, for they describe a faculty member who is both a teacher and a nurse. However, the relationship of faculty role identity to enhancement of students' clinical competencies is unclear.

REFERENCES

Ajzen, I., & Fishbein, M. *Understanding attitudes and predicting social behavior.* Englewood Cliffs, N.J.: Prentice-Hall, 1980.

Armington, C.L., Reinikka, E.A., & Creighton, H. Student evaluation — Threat or incentive? *Nursing Outlook,* 1972, *20,* 789-792.

Aspy, D. *Toward a technology for humanizing education.* Champaign, IL: Research Press, 1972.

Barham, V.Z. Identifying effective behavior of the nursing instructor through critical incidents. *Nursing Research,* 1965, *14,* 65-68.

Brodkorb, M.M. *Identification of the relative importance of selected instructional behaviors of clinical nursing faculty by undergraduate nursing students.* Unpublished master's thesis, University of Illinois at the Medical Center, 1979.

Brown, S.T. Faculty and student perceptions of effective clinical teachers. *Journal of Nursing Education,* 1981, *20*(9), 4-15.

Brunclik, H., Thurston, J.R., & Feldhusen, J. The empathy inventory. *Nursing Outlook,* 1967, *15,* 42-45.

Butler, C.B., & Geitgey, D.A. A tool for evaluating teachers. *Nursing Outlook,* 1970, *18,* 56-58.

Costin, F., Greenough, W.T., & Menges, R.J. Student ratings of college teaching: Reliability, validity, and usefulness. *Review of Educational Research,* 1971, *41,* 511-535.

Dixon, J.K., & Koerner, B. Faculty and student perceptions of effective classroom teaching in nursing. *Nursing Research,* 1976, *25,* 300-305.

Fishbein, M., & Ajzen, I. *Beliefs, attitudes, intentions, and behavior.* Reading, Mass.: Addison-Wesley, 1975.

Flanagan, J.C. The critical incident technique. *Psychological Bulletin,* 1954, *41,* 327-328.

Grebremedhin, N. *Opinions of second and fourth year baccalaureate nursing students about teacher qualities that facilitated their learning experiences.* Unpublished master's thesis, University of Washington, 1974.

Guthrie, E.R. The evaluation of teaching. *American Journal of Nursing,* 1953, *53,* 220-221.

Hassenplug, L.W. The good teacher. *Nursing Outlook,* 1965, *13,* 24-27.

Hawkins, J.W. *Clinical experiences in collegiate nursing education.* New York: Springer, 1981.

Heidgerken, L.E. *The nursing student evaluates her teachers.* Philadelphia: Lippincott, 1952.

Hook, C.M., & Rosenshine, B.V. Accuracy of teacher reports of their classroom behavior. *Review of Educational Research,* 1979, *49*(1), 1-12.

Infante, M.S. *The clinical laboratory in nursing education.* New York: Wiley, 1975.

Jackson, M.O. Instructor and course evaluation based on student-identified criteria. *Journal of Nursing Education,* 1977, *16*(2), 8-13.

Jacobson, M.D. Effective and ineffective behavior of teachers of nursing as described by their students. *Nursing Research,* 1966, *15,* 218-224.

Karns, P.J., & Schwab, T.A. Therapeutic communication and clinical instruction. *Nursing Outlook,* 1982, *30,* 39-43.

Kiker, M. Characteristics of the effective teacher. *Nursing Outlook,* 1973, *21,* 721-723.

Layton, M.M. How instructors' attitudes affect students. *Nursing Outlook,* 1969, *17,* 27-29.

Lowery, B.J., Keene, A.P., & Hyman, I.A. Nursing students' and faculty opinion of student evaluation of teachers. *Nursing Research,* 1971, *20,* 436-439.

Mannion, M. A taxonomy of instructional behaviors applicable to the guidance of learning activities in the clinical setting in baccalaureate nursing education (Doctoral dissertation, The Catholic University of America, 1968). *Dissertation Abstracts,* 1968, *29,* 4724B. (University Microfilms No. 60-09098).

McKay, R.P. Issues in graduate education: Training for education in teaching. *Journal of Nursing Education,* 1971, *10*(8), 11-20.

McLane, A.M. Core competencies of master's-prepared nurses. *Nursing Research,* 1978, *28,* 48-53.

Meleca, C.J., Schimpfhauser, F., Witteman, J.K., & Sachs, L. Clinical instruction in nursing: A national survey. *Journal of Nursing Education,* 1981, *20*(8), 32-40.

Menges, R.J. The new reporters: Students rate instruction. In C.R. Pace (Ed.), *Evaluating learning and teaching.* San Francisco: Jossey-Bass, 1973.

Menges, R.J. Evaluating teaching effectiveness: What is the proper role for students? *Liberal Education,* 1979, *65,* 356-369.

Mims, F.H. Students evaluate faculty. *Nursing Outlook,* 1970, *18,* 53-55.

O'Shea, H.S., & Parsons, M.K. Clinical instruction: Effective and ineffective teacher behaviors. *Nursing Outlook,* 1979, *27,* 411-415.

Pugh, E.J. Factors influencing congruence between beliefs, intentions, and behavior in the clinical teaching of nursing (Doctoral dissertation, Northwestern University, 1980). *Dissertation Abstracts International,* 1980, *41*(6), 2521A-2522A. (University Microfilms No. 8026902).

Pugh, E.J. Dynamics of teaching-learning interaction. *Nursing Forum,* 1976, *15*(1), 47-58.

Rauen, K.C. The clinical instructor as role model. *Journal of Nursing Education,* 1974, *13*(3), 33-40.

Stafford, L.F. Determining effective nursing teacher behaviors in clinical settings (Doctoral dissertation, Texas A & M University, 1978). *Dissertation Abstracts International,* 1979, *39*(7), 4154A. (University Microfilms No. 7901008).

Wood, V. Student evaluations of their tutors in four schools of nursing 1. *Nursing Times,* 1971a, *67,* 97-100.

Wood, V. Student evaluations of their tutors in four schools of nursing 2. *Nursing Times,* 1971a, *67,* 101-104.

Zasowska, M.A. A descriptive survey of significant factors in the clinical laboratory experience in baccalaureate education for nursing (Doctoral dissertation, Teachers College, Columbia University, 1967). *Dissertation Abstracts International,* 1967, *28,* 1951B (University Microfilms No. 67-12, 714).

Chapter Four:
Predicting Academic Success

Chapter Four:
Predicting Academic Success

Richard E. Grant, R.N., Ph.D.

Introduction

Nursing educators are concerned with being able to predict how students will perform. There is a desire to select the most highly qualified candidates for entry into the nursing major and send only the most skilled and devoted graduates into the community. In the past, a major concern was utilization of equitable and productive admission criteria because there were far more applicants for admission to the nursing major than places. In 1981, schools of nursing appeared to be experiencing a decline in enrollment (n.a., 1981) and there was a new danger of admitting larger numbers of less qualified applicants.

There are several reasons for wanting to predict academic success. There is a financial loss to the student and the community when the student withdraws prior to completion of a program. Those at risk for failure may receive special counseling if identified early. Students who have difficulty in completion of a program may effect the morale and achievement of other class members. The quality of instruction can be affected because faculty might believe they should teach to their slowest learners. There is always the possibility that some highly qualified candidates might not be admitted into a program because less qualified students have already been accepted. Finally, the student who must be dropped from a program because of academic difficulties can be affected psychologically.

This chapter focuses on the research of cognitive predictors of academic success. It is intended to serve as a resource guide. Readers interested in detailed aspects of a study are referred to the research without the need for an extensive literature search.

An excellent monograph by Franklin (1975) reviewed the work prior to 1975 and concluded,

> ...all this research can be confusing to the uninitiated for the authors are either inconclusive in their findings or contradict each other. The admissions officer who wishes to justify his position for or against selective admissions policies has enough evidence to support whatever stance he may take. In addition, the evidence which is available from research does not indicate that admission tests or any other single criterion can discriminate the successful from the unsuccessful student in college or in life, nor do the tests seem able to accomplish the fine discrimination required to predict which average student will succeed or fail. (p. 16)

She compared schools using selective admission criteria with schools not using them and found that there "was a significantly higher proportion of failures in nonselective schools than in selective schools" (p. 35). Also, a higher percentage of students withdrew from nonselective programs for academic reasons, while nearly an identical number withdrew from both types of programs for nonacademic reasons. The development of adequate predictors of academic success is important if nursing programs are to make the best use of scarce resources and to ensure that the largest number of students benefit from the investment.

An analysis of the literature from the past ten years revealed that studies can be categorized in three areas: (1) predicting achievement in the nursing major, (2) measuring success during the nursing major, and (3) predicting graduates' performance especially on the State Board Test Pool Examination, using pre-nursing and intra-nursing performance criteria.

Predicting Achievement in the Nursing Major

The diversity of the criteria used to select students with the highest chances for success in the nursing major illustrates several difficulties. The most widely accepted criteria are the most traditional. These are grade point average (GPA) from high school or from college work and scores obtained on admissions tests, e.g., PACE, ACT, SAT, and GRE. The most common criterion used for prediction is grade point average (GPA), although calculated a variety of ways. They range from the GPAs of specific course areas (e.g., science, math, social sciences) to cummulative GPAs from high school or college work. Stankovich (1977) compared the American College Test Program (ACT), high school biology grade, math grade, total high school GPA and final GPA for college work. She found that high school accumulative GPA was significant in predicting college success. Anatomy and physiology grades were also significantly related to how students performed in the nursing major. Stronck (1979) compared the predictive ability of GPA, various entrance examinations, and the use of interviews and letters of recommendation. He found that interviews and recommendation letters were of little value while GPA was the best predictor of future success.

Accumulative GPA and Graduate Record Examination (GRE) are the most common criteria used for entrance into graduate nursing education. Three studies are reported which examine the predictive ability of these criteria. Thomas (1977) found both criteria to be good predictors with the provision that not all students should be treated as a single class, as students choosing different areas of concentration (i.e., medical-surgical, nursing of children, nursing service administration, and psychiatric nursing) scored differently on the variables measured. Ainslie et al. (1976) analyzed GPA, GRE, age, and number of years since subjects received their baccalaureate degrees. They found only weak association on all variables except age which was of no value. Thomas (1974) found that the verbal section of the GRE and GPA were both significant predictors. She qualified her results when she stated,

> ... the status of the art of predicting success in nursing education raises more questions than it answers. Certainly, the relatively small variance explained by the predictors would preclude the rigid use of test scores or baccalaureate GPA level to make admission decisions. Rather, support is provided for the practice of flexibility in admission policies. (pp. 159)

Montgomery and Palmer (1976) examined the predictive abilities of the ACT scores, earned college credit hours, age, and whether or not the subject had taken high school chemistry and/or physics. They found that ACT scores correlated with academic achievement and that the best predictors were age of subject and number of college credits earned. Older students with more credits did better.

Bello (1977) found that age, reading ability, high school algebra grades and college science grades were the best predictors of nursing GPA. She recommended increased selectivity in admissions emphasizing that reading ability and supportive remedial services be stressed to assist students to succeed. Yess (1979) compared the SAT scores and high school GPA as predictors of nursing GPA. He found that the predictors which consistently accounted for variance in college GPA were high school English average, and the SAT Verbal and Math subscores.

A wide variety of other measures have been examined for predictive ability. Willett et al. (1971) examined the College Qualification Tests (CQT), Forrer Structured Sentence Completion Test (FSSCT), General Information Questionnaire (GIQ), Raven's progressive Matrices (Ravens), Minnesota Multiphasic Personality Inventory (MMPI), and the Sixteen Personality Factor Questionnaire (16PF). They found that the CQT was the best predictor of academic achievement with the 16PF a next predictor. The CQT evaluated for academic factors and the 16PF assessed personality factors for success. They suggest that pre-entrance selection procedures reduce dropout rates and may have high value.

Seither (1974) studied the California Short Form Test of Mental Maturity, the California Test of Personality, and the California Reading Test. Only reading comprehension was related to nursing GPA. Tracy and Baer (1979) evaluated the Structure of Intellect Test (SOI) and concluded that the test is a useful instrument in determining patterns of intellectual abilities necessary for success in some professions, including nursing.

Lamoureaux and Johannsen (1977) used the George Washington University Nursing Test, the Strong-Campbell Interest Inventory, the Coopersmith Self-Esteem Inventory, the Cattel 16PF Personality Test, and two investigator developed questionnaires to examine student persistence/non-persistence in nursing education. While no test singularly was highly predictive, a subset of variables were correlated with the criterion variable. These were the Strong-Campbell Registered Nurse Scale (standardized score), the George Washington University Nursing Test (raw score), Nelson Denny Test (raw score), whether the student was employed before entering the program, the number of miles traveled to school (one way), the Adolph Whaler Index, and the Cattel 16PF Forthright-Astute scale (raw score). Their work demonstrated the complex nature of the study of academic success.

Singh (1972) examined the Ravens Test, the Mill-Hill Vocabulary Test, and Haward's Reading Comprehension Test to determine if reading ability was a better indicator of future success than the more traditional criteria. Reading comprehension was unrelated to which students would complete the program. Smith and Pervanser (1975), on the other hand, reported that reading ability and GPA were highly correlated.

Burgess et al. (1972) found that the pre-nursing GPA was consistently a good predictor of nursing GPA. Clemence and Brink (1978) question the predictive ability of any kind of pre-admissions test criteria on the basis that such tests do not truly measure performance potential, rather past performance successes.

A few conclusions seem warranted. First, the best predictor of future success is past success. The traditional criteria used for selection of students which rely on past demonstrated achievement are most predictive of nursing GPA. They do not, however, suggest those factors which predict which students will complete their nursing education. The situation may be one where highly complex inter-relationships between intellectual ability, personality variables, and teacher-student interactions determine whether students will succeed and finish their nursing education. Continuing effort needs to be put into the multi-variate approach in research to answer our questions.

Measuring Success during the Nursing Major

One trend that emerges from the literature measuring student performance is that educators are seeking instruments that measure more than the ability to recall factual knowledge and perform rote skills. Evaluation is increasingly focused on patient care as the standard of measurement with education viewed as a means to that end. Because of societal issues over the past two decades, much of this effort has been devoted to measuring how ethnic minorities and the educationally disadvantaged perform and how they can be assisted to improve their performance in nursing programs. This effort is also a result of the rapid growth of Associate Degree programs.

Moore and Pentecost (1979) studied educationally disadvantaged students in California. They were concerned about the large numbers of students reapplying for admission in spite of the fact that they had "overwhelming grade point deficiencies" (p. 51). They identified four major areas where students in nursing need advisement: scheduling, finances, personal needs and expectations, and basic academic skills. They developed a comprehensive support system for these applicants which included an orientation workshop, tutoring, prescriptive learning assistance, and personal counseling and academic advisement. Evaluation of the project resulted in statistical support that the program had prevented course failure and attrition of students whose admission academic profiles would have predicted failure.

Huckabay (1979) used formative evaluations to study the effect of grading on the development of mastery over selected content in a graduate nursing program. Using one experimental and two control groups, she tested the effects of grading (experimental group, N=25); learning by lecture-discussion without grading (N=32); and learning by formative evaluation without grading (N=35). Findings from the study indicate that the teaching strategy "that implements without grading will be most successful" (p. 177). Furthermore, she suggests that grading may act as an inhibitor to learning.

Owen and Feldhusen (1970) compared the effectiveness of three models of multi-variate prediction for academic success in identifying the criterion variance of achievement in nursing education. The first model used first semester grade average in an attempt to predict subsequent semester scores. The second used each semester average, including the grade points from previous semester scores. There was rapid drift away from the first semester grade point so that one could not predict the last semester GPA from the first (Model I). The second model, a continuously accumulative grade point, enabled the researchers to most accurately predict subsequent semesters.

Reviewing the research on intra-nursing success is difficult because the material is so diverse. Increasing emphasis is placed on early identification of stumbling blocks for students with group or individual counseling to assist the students to complete school.

Predicting Graduates Performance

Most of the research on predicting graduate performance relates to how well students perform on State Board Test Pool Examinations (SBTPE). Questions relate to whether student performance on tests or class grades is predictive of SBTPE performance. Muhlenkamp (1971) examined SAT, Engligh test scores, grades for specific nursing courses and a developmental psychology course, seventh semester GPA, and the NLN Achievement Test scores to determine if they correlated significantly with performance on SBTPEs. She found that the seventh semester GPA had the highest correlation for most of the State Board section scores. The NLN Natural Science Exam was the second best predictor.

Nursing Outlook (1971) reported that for one Associate Degree program, the NLN Examination on Maternal and Child Nursing was the best predictor of how students would perform on the SBTPEs. Because of the small sample of students (N=23), and that only one school was included, it was recommended that it be replicated using a large number of students from a variety of schools. Beckman and Steindler (1971) reported on a similar study at a collegiate nursing program, using the Wechsler Adult Intelligence Scale (WAIS), SAT, and high school rank. These were correlated with college GPA and the results of SBTPE scores. It was found that the SAT Verbal Test score had the highest correlation. Verbal or reading ability appeared to be the critical factor for success.

Bell and Martindill (1975) also used the NLN Achievement tests. They found that the Nursing of Children and Obstetric Nursing tests had the highest correlations with SBTPE results. They concluded, however, that the State Board Examinations measure common abilities rather than independent ones. Their results suggest that nursing programs should develop and validate prediction equations to assist nurses in preparing for the SBTPEs. Deardorff, Denner and Miller (1976) followed the Bell and Martindill suggestion by designing predictor equations based on NLN Achievement Tests used as sets. SBTPE scores were subject to stepwise multiple regression analysis and it was found that the equations as applied were successful in predicting the SBTPE scores of their subjects. They again found that, while the NLN Achievement Tests and the SBTPEs appear to be content specific, all tests contain overlap which may be of more importance than currently recognized. Their major recommendation was that the predictive character of the NLN Examinations be used for guiding students who are preparing to take SBTPEs.

Washburn (1980) studied the relationship between the NLN Achievement Tests and the SBTPEs with a group of 166 graduates of a diploma program. She found highly significant correlations for all tests, with the best predictor being the NLN Nursing Care of Patients II Achievement Test. Shelley, Kannamer and Raile (1976) correlated NLN Achievement Test scores and selected course grades with SBTPE scores. They found that, while some course grades (i.e., Fundamentals of Nursing, Zoology, Microbiology, and Chemistry) did significantly correlate with SBTPE scores, a much higher correlation was established with the NLN Examinations. They concluded that NLN Achievement Tests should continue to be used as indicators of how students will perform on SBTPEs and that they be used for advising students.

Perez (1977) compared ACT, GPAs at various academic levels, GPAs for science and social science prerequisite courses and NLN Achievement Test scores with scores obtained on SBTPEs. She found that the ACT Social Science Reading score, GPA at the end of the freshman year, and the social science accumulative grade point were fairly good predictors. General reading ability was the most important factor in influencing how students performed. NLN scores were not significant.

Wolfe and Bryant (1973) studied NLN Achievement Test scores and found that about 75% of scores were achieved as a result of nursing education and that about 25% came from other education or life experiences. Eighty percent of the scores related to mastery of subject matter with two major exceptions. Psychiatric Nursing and Pediatric Nursing scores apparently result from a wide variety of experiences including education, which assist students to "adapt, adjust, and deal with individuals and situations" (p. 314). The study developed a causal model for determination of those factors which produce different levels of performance on the NLN Achievement Tests and the SBTPEs.

Cusick and Harckham (1973) studied six personality variables used in admissions decisions as predictors of success on SBTPEs. They found that the scales: achievement, orderliness, persistence, congeniality, altruism, and respectfulness were not related to success on examinations.

Outtz (1979) used high school GPA, high school science GPA, SAT, and college science GPA in an attempt to find predictors for success on SBTPEs for black nursing students. She found a significant correlation between high school and college GPAs, but the college accumulative GPA seemed to be the best predictor of success on SBTPEs, followed by the SAT Verbal Test. Again, verbal or reading ability was found to be a key factor.

Aquino, Trent, and Deutsch (1979) examined SBTPE performance of foreign nurse graduates. They used the State-Trait Inventory, the Test of English as a Foreign Language, and five achievement tests in two formats; short answer and multiple choice. They found that test format did not affect performance. This sample of foreign nurses lacked the knowledge in specific areas of pediatric nursing content. Test anxiety did not appear to play as much of a role as generally assumed. It is interesting that beyond the fact that the subjects lacked knowledge in one specific area, their scores were significantly correlated with reading ability.

Two studies predicted job performance. Dubs (1975) investigated the relationships among on-the-job performance of graduates from a diploma school of nursing, school achievement, and State Board scores. She found that the accumulative grade point averages and nursing theory grades were the best predictors of success on SBTPEs, while nursing practice grades were the best predictors of on-the-job performance.

Wilson (1975) studied the job performance of 153 graduates of an Associate Degree program. Results indicated that there was no significant relationship between measures of scholastic success (i.e., GPA, and State Board scores) and the rated job performance.

Conclusions and Recommendations

The research devoted to establishing definitive admissions criteria continues to be confusing and conflicting. It is likely that the critical variables beyond prior achievement which enable a student to succeed in the nursing major, and which can be measured prior to admission, have not been clearly identified. One exception may be reading skill. While there seems little doubt that future success is dependent upon multi-variate phenomena, it seems of little value to continue documenting that past success is a good predictor of future success. However, with the redefinition of the national licensing examination, it may be necessary to replicate some of these findings. Research efforts ought to be devoted to examining those aspects of curricula and teaching-learning processes which contribute to high level nursing care.

REFERENCES

Ainslie, N., Andersen, L., Colby, B., Hoffman, M., Meserve, K., O'Connor, C. & Ouimet, K. Predictive value of selected admission criteria for graduate nursing education. *Nursing Research*, 1976, *25*(4), 296-299.

Aquino, N., Trent, P. & Deutsch, J. Factors related to foreign nurse graduates' test-taking performance. *Nursing Research*, 28(2), 111-114.

Araneta, N. & Miller, C. Philosophical systems of weighting clinical performance in nursing. *International Journal for Nursing Studies*, 1970, *7*(4), 235-424.

Backman, M. & Steindler, F. Let's examine: Prediction of achievement in a collegiate nursing program and performance on State Board Examinations. *Nursing Outlook*, 1971, *19*(7), 487.

Bell, J. & Martindill, C. A cross-validation study for predictors of scores on State Board Examinations. *Nursing Research*, 1976, *25*(1), 54-57.

Bello, A. *Factors which predict success or failure in an associate degree nursing program.* Bureau of Occupational and Adult Education (DHEW/OE), Washington, D.C.

Bendall, E. The learning process in student nurses. *Nursing Times*, 1971, *67*(44), 173-175.

Bower, F. Normative or criterion-referenced evaluation? *Nursing Outlook*, 1974, *22*(8), 499-502.

Bower, F. Relation of the learning environment to ethnic minority achievement in a nursing curriculum. *Communicating Nursing Research*, January 1976, 205-224.

Burgess, M., Duffy, M. & Temple F. Two studies of prediction of success in a collegiate program of nursing. *Nursing Research*, 1972,*21*(4), 357-366.

Clemence, B. & Brink, P. How predictive are admissions criteria? *Journal of Nursing Education*, 1978, *17*(4), 5-10.

Coetsee, M. *The Prediction of Academic Success in Baccalaureate Nursing Students.* Unpublished Doctoral dissertation (D.S.N.), University of Alabama, Birmingham, 1979.

Connors, V. *The Prediction of State Board Test Pool Examination Scores from National League for Nursing Achievement Test Scores and Academic Indices.* Unpublished Doctoral dissertation (Ed.D.), University of Houston, Texas, 1979.

Cusick, P. & Harckham, L. *The Effectiveness of Six Personality Variables in Predicting Success on the Nursing State Board Examination.* Research in Education, July, 1973.

Cyrs, R. Performance objectives: The unending controversy. *Journal of Practical Nursing,* 1976, *26*(11), 33-34, 37, 41.

Deardorff, M., Denner, P. & Miller, C. Selected National League for Nursing Achievement scores as predictors of State Board Examination scores. *Nursing Research,* 1976 *25*(1), 35-38.

Debarbrie, M. *Factors Associated with the Prediction of Success in an Educational Program for Licensed Vocational Nurses.* Unpublished Doctoral dissertation (Ph.D.), University of Texas, Austin, 1972.

Di-Marco, N., Norton, S. & Fendler, D. Predictors of practical Nursing State Board Examination scores. *International Journal for Nursing Studies,* 1979, *16*(1), 59-63.

Dubs, R. Comparison of student achievement with performance ratings of graduates and State Board Examination scores. *Nursing Research,* 1975, *24*(1), 59-62, 64.

Dyer, M. The concepts of evaluation as related to the total curriculum, individual courses, and students. *NLN Publications, No. 16-1418,* 1970, 8-21.

Franklin, E. Selective and nonselective admissions criteria in junior college nursing programs. *League Exchange,* 1975, (104), 1-68.

Frederickson, K. & Mayer, G. Problem solving skills: What effect does education have? *American Journal of Nursing,* 1977, *77*(7), 1167-1169.

Frejlach, G. & Corcoran, S. Measuring clinical performance. *Nursing Outlook,* 1971, *19*(4), 270-271.

Harrison, O. & Hoffmeister, J. A statistical method for development of subconcepts in nursing. *Nursing Research,* 1977, *26*(6), 448-451.

Hayter, J. An approach to laboratory evaluation. *Journal of Nursing Education,* 1973, *12*(4), 17-22.

Huckabay, L. Cognitive-affective consequences of grading versus nongrading of formative evaluations. *Nursing Research,* 1979, *28*(3), 173-178.

Jones, C.W. Models for Predicting Academic Success and State Board *Scores for Associate Degree Nursing Students.* Unpublished Doctoral dissertation (Ed.D.), Illinois State University, Jacksonville, 1977.

Kramer, M. & Cowles, J. Weighting and distributing course grades. *Nursing Outlook,* 1974, *22*(3), 176-179.

Krumme, U. The case for criterion-referenced measurement. *Nursing Outlook,* 1975, *23*(12), 764-770.

Lamoureaux, M. & Johannsen, C. Multiple criteria development for the selection community college nursing program students. *Research in Education,* April, 1979.

Landureth, L. & Lameddola, J. Education and the hospital: Computers in nursing education. *Hospitals,* 1973, *47*(5), 99-100.

Layton, J. Students select their own grades. *Nursing Outlook,* 1972, *20*(5), 327-329.

Lycon, A. *The Prediction of Academic Achievement of Pre-Nursing and Nursing Students by Using Attitudinal and Preferential Methods.* Unpublished Doctoral dissertation (Ph.D.), North Texas State University, Denton, 1980.

Marriner, A. Student self-evaluation and the contracted grade. *Nursing Forum*, 1974, *13*(2), 130-135.

Melcolm, N., Venn, R. & Bausell, R. The prediction of State Board Test Pool Examinations scores within an integrated curriculum. *Journal of Nursing Education*, 1981, *20*(5), 24-28.

Merrill, L. *Field Dependence Independence as Related to Selected Career Decisions and Predictors of Academic Success in Nursing.* Unpublished Doctoral dissertation (Ph.D.), University of Nebraska, Lincoln, 1978.

Mims, R., Yeaworth, R. & Hornstein, S. Effectiveness of an interdisciplinary course in human sexuality. *Nursing Research*, 1974, *23*(3), 248-253.

Montgomery, J. & Palmer, P. Reducing attrition in an AD program. *Nursing Outlook*, 1971, *24*(1), 49-52.

Moore, B. & Pentecost, W. CSULB nursing: Educationally disadvantaged students can succeed. *Journal of Nursing Education*, 1979, *18*(6), 50-58.

Muhlenkamp, A. Prediction of State Board scores in a baccalaureate program. *Nursing Outlook*, 1971, *19*(1), 57.

Oliver, W., Ambrosino, R. & Rorabaush, S. Special trauma training for nurses in hospital emergency departments. *Health Service Representative*, 1974, *89*(2), 112-118.

Outtz, J. Predicting the success on State Board Examinations for blacks. *Journal of Nursing Education*, 1979, *18*(9), 25-40.

Owen, S. & Feldhusen, J. *Using Performance Data Gathered at Several Stages of Achievement in Predicting Subsequent Performance.* Research in Education, November, 1970.

Paduano, M. Evaluation in the nursing laboratory: An honest appraisal. *Nursing Outlook*, 1974, *22*(11), 702-705.

Papcum, I. Results of achievement tests and State Board tests in an Associate Degree program. *Nursing Outlook*, 1971, *19*(5), 341.

Perez, T. Investigation of academic moderator variables to predict success on State Board of Nursing Examinations in a baccalaureate nursing program. *Journal of Nursing Education*, 1977, *16*(8), 16-23.

Pierson, L. *The Development of Academic Success Prediction Equations for use in The Selection and Advisement of Student Nurses in an Associate Degree Nursing Program.* Unpublished Doctoral dissertation (Ed.D.), Brigham Young University, Provo, Utah, 1975.

Pontious, S. *Multi-variate Prediction of Academic Achievement in a Collegiate Program of Nursing.* Unpublished Doctoral dissertation (Ph.D.), New Mexico State University, Socorro, 1980.

Reed, C. & Feldhusen, J. State Board Examination score prediction for Associate Degree Nursing Program graduates. *Nursing Research*, 1972, *21*(2), 149-153.

Richards, E. Use of the computer in evaluation. *NLN Publications, No. 16-1687*, 1977, 134-138.

Schwirian, P. *Prediction of Successful Nursing Performance*. Research in Education, July, 1978.

Seither, F.F. Prediction of achievement in baccalaureate nursing education. *Journal of Nursing Education*, 1980, *19*(3), 28-36.

Seither, F.F. A predictive validity study of screening measures used to select practical nursing students. *Nursing Research*, 1974, *23*(1), 60-63.

Sime, A. Prediction of success in a Master's Degree program in nursing. *Psychological Reports*, 1978, *42*(3, pt. 1), 783-799.

Shelley, B., Kennamer, E. & Raile, M. Correlation of NLN Achievement Test scores with State Board Test Pool Examination scores. *Nursing Outlook*, 1976, *24*(1), 52-55.

Singh, A. The predictive value of cognitive tests for selection of pupil nurses. *Nursing Times*, 1972, *68*(23), 89-92.

Smith, D. & Pervanser, J. Reading, a major finding in determining success in nursing education. *Reading Horizons*, 1974, *14*(3), 125-127.

Stankovich, M. *The Statistical Predictability of the Academic Performance of Registered Nursing Students at Macomb*. Research in Education, March, 1979.

Stein, R. The Graduate Record Examination: Does it predict performance in nursing programs? *The Nurse Educator*, 1978, *3*(4), 16-19.

Stephens, K. Real examinations — a new perspective on nursing evaluations. *NLN Publications, No. 16-1538*, 1975, 163-171.

Stronck, D. Predicting student performance from college admission criteria. *Nursing Outlook*, 1979, *27*(9), 604-607.

Tatham, E. *Nursing and Dental Hygiene Selection Procedures. Part 2: An Examination of Academic Variables as Predictors of Success*. Research in Education, August, 1976.

Thomas, B. Prediction of success in graduate nursing administration program. *Nursing Research*, 1974, *23*(2), 156-159.

Tracy, G. & Baer, M. *Correlating Intellectual Abilities with Successful Vocation Training and Placement of Licensed Practical Nurses Using the Structure of Intellect Assessment Procedure*. Louisiana State Department of Education, Baton Rouge, 1979.

Vashchenko, M. & Napnenko, E. Predictors of success in health visiting. *Nursing Times*, 1973, 1b269(14), 57-60.

Willett, E., Riffel, P., Breen, L. & Dickson, E. Selection and success of students in a hospital School of Nursing. *Canadian Nurse*, 1971, *67*(1), 41-45.

Wilson, B. *Evaluation and Prediction of Rated Job Performance of Nursing Graduates*. Health Resources Administration (DHEW/PHS), Bethesda, Maryland. Division of Nursing, 1975.

Wolfe, L. & Bryant, L. A causal model of nursing education and State Board Examination scores. *Nursing Research*, 1978, *27*(5), 311-315.

PREDICTING ACADEMIC SUCCESS

Yess, J. *Predicting the Academic Success of Community College Students in Specific Programs of Study*. Research in Education, November, 1979.

n.a. The interpretation of scores on the NLN Pre-Admission and Classification Examination. *Nursing Outlook*, 1970, *18*(12), 47.

n.a. The interpretation of scores on the NLN Pre-Admission and Classification Examination. *Nursing Outlook*, 1971, *19*(5), 341.

n.a. *Health Personnel Manpower Study*. U.S. Government Printing Office, Washington, D.C., 1981.

Chapter Five:
Stress of the Returning
R.N. Student

Chapter Five:
Stress of the Returning R.N. Student

Pamela A. Baj, R.N., M.S.

The purpose of this chapter is to examine the issue of stress experienced by Registered Nurse (R.N.) students enrolled in baccalaureate programs. Ultimately implications for research will be developed which will demonstrate the relationship between the phenomenon of stress and the characteristics of the R.N. student as an adult learner.

The Present Situation

A review of the literature indicates that a discrepancy exists between the stated ideals of nursing leadership and the reality of its membership with respect to the credentials attained for entry at the practice level (Balogh, 1970; Woolley, 1978; Muzio, 1979; Styles, 1982). At present in the United States there are 958,308 R.N.'s working in nursing but 722,861 (75.4%) have less than a baccalaureate as their highest academic credential (ANA, 1981). The ANA's 1978 resolutions on "entry into practice" mandate two categories of nursing practice by 1985. The resolutions call for professional nursing to require baccalaureate preparation and technical nursing to require associate degree level or equivalent preparation. Each category would receive distinct titles, competencies, and (by implication) rewards and responsibilities (ANA, 1978).

Driven by historical imperative, economic necessity, chance opportunity, or genuine desire to broaden their knowledge and competency, increasing numbers of R.N.'s are returning to school to obtain the baccalaureate credential (Hillsmith, 1978). While some leaders anticipated a temporary pool of applicants which would abate after five years (de Tornyay, 1979), current statistics would indicate otherwise. First, despite future intentions, at the present time no state laws require a baccalaureate credential as minimum requirement for entry into practice (Styles, 1982). Second, of the 1389 programs in the United States that prepare for R.N. licensure, only 368 are generic baccalaureate programs, while 333 hospital diploma and 688 associate degree programs operate (NLN, 1980). Recent developments such as the closure of Skidmore College's 60-year-old baccalaureate program and the trustee proposal at Duke University to replace a baccalaureate and retrenched graduate program with an associate degree program (AJN News, 1982) would seem to indicate that nurses will continue to acquire less than a baccalaureate credential as their first credential for some future time. It is likely that the pool of potential R.N. applicants to baccalaureate programs will continue to rise.

Review of the Literature

The literature has reflected the movement of the R.N. student back to school (Badossi, 1980; Balogh, 1970; Banertscher, 1979; Boddie, 1970; Choinski, 1978; "Diploma schools," 1980; Galliford, 1970; Hillsmith 1978; La Violette, 1979; McGettigan, 1970; McKay, 1978; MacMaster, 1979; Muzio, 1979: Nyquist, 1973; Rosenstein, 1978; Shane, 1980; Styles, 1982; Tourneau, 1970; Wilson, 1978; Woolley, 1978). It is unclear whether or not the schools were expecting the tensions that developed as the R.N. student was introduced into the baccalaureate programs. Many articles have loosely described the R.N. student enrolled in the B.S.N. program (Balogh, 1970; Boddie, 1970; Hillsmith, 1978; Muzio, 1979; Shane, 1980; Wilson, 1978; Woolley, 1978; Zorn, 1980). Of the approximately 120,000 baccalaureate nursing students enrolled today, about 16% are R.N.'s seeking a baccalaureate degree and roughly two out of three of these R.N.'s are enrolled in generic baccalaureate programs (ANA, 1981).

Experiences such as those reported by Woolley (1978) are unsettling: one-third of an entering group of R.N. students dropped out due to academic performance, ill health, personal crises, and a general disillusionment with the program. Similar disaffection was noted by other authors (Wilson, 1978; Shane, 1980). Although suggesting that the problem was complex, most writing in this area remains anecdotal, descriptive, not well grounded in theoretical frameworks nor substantiated by research findings.

Hillsmith (1978) conducted a questionnaire survey of 119 R.N. students at the University of Bridgeport in 1976-1977. The primary purpose was to ascertain the motivation behind the R.N. student's return to school. While hinting at the existence of such stressors as finances, work schedules, and lack of familial support, the main thrust of the paper was the recognition of the attitude common to the R.N. respondents: "The insistence that one *is* a professional while, at the same time one is pursuing the degree which labels one 'professional' leads to a very definite ambivalence" (Hillsmith, 1978, p. 100). There are suggestions that differences in student self-perceptions and faculty opinions of R.N. students may be involved: "I greatly resent being told I can't hold a position (head nurse, supervisor) without the BSN when I have proven myself capable of performing the duties that go with that position" (Hillsmith, 1978, p. 101).

A similar anecdotal approach from the faculty perspective was presented by Woolley (1978). She basically saw the source of students' anxieties and tensions as a problem in socialization and role change: "We felt that the major cause of the anxiety was not amenable to change in our methods or the curriculum, but needed to be resolved by the students as they coped with the changes they were experiencing" (p. 104). Woolley noted that the students "place a high value on their experience" (p. 103) and yet the program was designed "to effect the changes required and prevent reinforcement of traditional behaviors by keeping students out of the hospital setting: all of their clinical nursing experience takes place with the community" (p. 104). After identifying the high value the students place on their previous professional experience, the faculty made a conscious decision to force the students into a situation where they had no previous experience and would become novices. Further discussion in the article was restricted to speculation on various socialization models for which no supporting data were presented.

Wilson (1978) conducted in-depth interviews with R.N. students collected as a theoretical sample of students withdrawing from a baccalaureate program. She identified a phase of adjustment and assessment on the student's part which was critical to the student's continuation of the program. As part of this phase, she identified the matching process, "a match between what the program is selling and what the nursing student is buying. Central to this exchange is the student's perception of what the nursing program is offering and how she views herself" (p. 439). Wilson also noted that another "matching" area concerned the student expectations of the teaching strategies and courses. The student's personal capabilities were also acknowledged to have impact on their matching process, however, there is a paucity of data to support these conclusions. These interview findings were not related to a larger theoretical framework.

A significant article on the subject of R.N. baccalaureate students was authored by Muzio and Ohashi (1979), which is a thoughtful challenge to the appropriateness of the generic model for R.N. students. Although the article is wholly expository (redundant), it does identify several special aspects of the problem. The authors question "whether the standards, program objectives, and educational processes and structures originally developed for generic students are appropriate for the RN group" (p. 528). The three characteristics of the R.N. group which were identified as affecting learning are: 1) prior knowledge and patterns of thought, 2) previous socialization, and 3) variations in age and life stage (Muzio & Ohashi, 1979). Unfortunately the authors assumed that R.N. students are concrete thinkers, somehow frozen in their intellectual development. The authors follow the model of Piaget, suggesting students must undergo a period of physical manipulation of objects, repeating the experience until the student can generalize the experience to abstract thought, the formal operational stage. Piaget's theories revolve largely around learning in children and may not be appropriate for adult learners (Kidd, 1977) but the emphasis on the cognitive aspects of the learning process in connection with the R.N. student is raised by the article.

Muzio and Ohashi do recognize the experiential knowledge acquired by R.N. students and the faculty's inability to fully evaluate this ability. The authors attribute this to the R.N. students' inability to verbalize this prior experience but do not further address the problem of evaluation. The process of self-actualization as advanced by Maslow (1971) is suggested as the primary motivation for the return of the R.N. student to the B.S.N. program, but no data are presented to support this. When contrasted with generic students, R.N. students were identified as advanced in age and concerned with different issues relating to maturity and adult development. The authors speculate that as adult learners the R.N. students tend to be interested in specific areas of knowledge or practice rather than general entry level roles. The paper concludes:

> Although little research-based information describing the differences between RNs and non-RNs in baccalaureate programs exists, we cannot ignore the preponderance of information from adult development, adult education, and social theory that indicates the reality of these differences (p.532).

In summary, the nursing literature indicates that the R.N. students may encounter a fair amount of stress in the B.S.N. program, reflected in attrition and perhaps hesitancy to enroll in such programs. In addition there are hints that the R.N. student presents special problems as an experienced, adult learner whose perceptions of herself may differ markedly from those of nursing educators. Although the suggestion is inferred that there is a link between the characteristics of the R.N. student as an adult learner and their self-perceptions and levels of stress, there is no research data to support or deny this connection at the present. These studies are summarized in Table 1.

TABLE 1

RESEARCH STUDIES ON RN STUDENTS RETURNING TO SCHOOL

Study	Description	Variables	Findings
Brown (1960)	Studied values change of RN's returning to school.	Values	Values of Returning RN's are more resistant to change.
Meyer (1960)	Studied graduate nurses returning to school	Values	Findings suggest little change in values of RN's returning to school.
Gortner (1968)	Nursing majors in 12 western universities surveyed. Study compared RN students to senior nursing in a baccalaureate program.	Values, personalities, educational and professional motivations, and socioeconomics.	RN students have a greater professional orientation; groups did not differ in personality; RN's came from families with lower socioeconomic positions.
Mullendore (1974)	44 RN Students in a baccalaureate program compared with associate degree students in determining interrelationships of self-esteem and internal-external locus of control with marital status, age, and academic achievement.	Self-esteem and locus of control.	RN's had a high measure of self-esteem.
Hillsmith (1976)	119 RN's at the University of Connecticut questioned why they were returning to school.	Reasons for returning to school for BS Degree.	Reasons: Achieve personal satisfaction, better job opportunities, professional growth and competence.
Wilson (1978)	Studied why RN students drop out.	Factors relevant to attrition.	Changed roles, academic or clinical requirements.
Glass (1981)	Studied professional socialization of RN students in second step programs.	Professional socialization	No significant findings.
Mallory (1982)	Studied possible outcome differences in scores received by Associate degree RN students and Diploma RN students returning for the BSN in generic and second step programs.	Outcome differences in NLN Achievement Tests.	RN graduates of generic and second step BSN programs are not significantly different in knowledge and application as measured by NLN Baccalaureate Level Achievement Tests.

Theoretical Frameworks

Three specific areas are identified by consideration of this literature on R.N. student stress. These areas are:

1) the nature and definition of stress — How is the term used? What are the parameters to be considered? How does the term relate to R.N. students?

2) the concepts of role stress and role strain — How do these terms of socialization relate to the R.N. student enrolled in a baccalaureate curriculum?

3) The process of adult learning — What is the process by which adults learn? What characteristics of R.N. students make them adult learners?

Each of these three areas will be discussed in order to show the potential interdependence of the self-perceptions of the R.N. students, their experiences as special adult learners, and their levels of stress in the baccalaureate program.

Concepts of Stress

Historically the term stress has been applied to mean at various times both stress as stimulus and stress as response to stimulus (Mason, 1975). Selye is originator of the modern concept of stress, growing from his studies on the General Adaptation Syndrome which is the triad of adrenal hypertrophy, thymic involution, and gastric ulceration he described in laboratory animals subjected to noxious stimuli.

Originally envisioned as a nonspecific response of physiology, Mason (1975), and others have established that confounding variables in the neuroendocrine system have misled earlier investigators. In reality, the responses of the neuroendocrine system are varied and specific and are capable of responding to a broad category of psychological stimuli termed arousal.

Selye (1974) has recently modified his earlier generalist, nonspecific, noncognitive view by suggesting that stress may be harmful (distress) or beneficial (eustress). This would appear to recognize the importance of mediating psychological influences. But the psychological approach to stress has evolved along different pathways as well.

Two major directions in the psychological interpretation of stress have been developed: the psychoanalytic approach personified by Vaillant (1977) and others and the cognitive appraisal perspective whose chief proponent is Lazarus (1978). The psychoanalysts view stress through the mediating processes (coping) and the patterns of individual behavior (adaptation). They see coping as a set of defense mechanisms which are *a priori* classified as beneficial or pathogenic. The outcome then depends on which defense mechanism is selected. Mason (1975) and others have pointed out that the confusion of values and context with the process of coping leads this approach astray. For instance, what may be ineffective, pathological denial for an individual in one setting may be effective and protective in another, although the same mechanism is employed in both instances.

Lazarus (1978) described the evolution of the understanding of the stress concept over a thirty-year time frame. For example, stress was used interchangeably with anxiety as a major source of pathological modes of adaptation (psychoanalytic view), a sort of intrapsychic pain which was used to explain behavior as tension-reducing and therefore self-reinforcing. However, two trends evolved in psychology which Lazarus (1978) credits with a more appropriate usage of the term.

First there was a movement from normative research, where large populations were studied to derive common elements of descriptive behavior, to ipsative research which emphasized individual characteristics and differences. The second trend was the rise of cognitive process in the explanation of human behavior. Lazarus (1978) states,

> For example, whereas in 1950 coping was almost universally viewed as a product of emotion and emotion viewed as a drive, my colleagues and I press the argument that emotions (and stress) are products of cognition, that is, of the way a person appraises or construes his or her relationship with the environment (p. 5).

The role of perception and appraisal are noteworthy. The idea that stress evolves out of one's own perception of the environment and one's relationship with the environment is critical to understanding the concept of stress.

There have been three variations in the attempt to define stress as a problem of stimulus and response (Lazarus & Launier, 1978). The first view is that stress refers to some stimulus, a force directed at a system which will provoke a change. The second view is that stress refers to the response of the system to the stimulus, i.e., the provoked change. The third view is that stress refers to the process or relationship of any individual system to its environment.

Lazarus (1978) has termed this relationship a transaction to emphasize two important aspects. One, the relationship between person and environment or between two variables is not uni-directional but a two-way approach and probably multi-directional. Secondly, the use of the word transaction implies a simultaneous modification of both person and environment in a mutually dependent fashion. This transactional nature of stress bears special emphasis.

The level of the system under consideration also needs to be considered in defining stress. As a hierarchy of systems man can be analyzed on various levels: cultural, social, psychological, cellular, or molecular (Mason, 1975). For general purposes of discussing stress, Lazarus (1978) identifies three broad areas: social, psychological and physiological. Although the three levels unquestionably interrelate with one another, one needs to consider which level is the subject of discussion in any particular situation. For instance, although psychological forces may affect somatic responses, it is inappropriate to use physiological stress measures to index psychological stress since "the same somatic response could have many non-psychological causes" (Lazarus, 1978, p. 17). This aspect of stress may be described as its multi-level nature and must be kept in mind when stress is being measured or described in any subject.

Measuring Cognitive Psychosocial Stress: Inherent Problems

Stress is defined by Lazarus (1980) as "any event in which environmental or internal demands (or both) tax or exceed the adaptive resources of an individual, social system, or tissue system" (p. 96). Within Lazarus' framework of stress, special problems inherent in measuring or quantifying stress in general and R.N. baccalaureate students in particular become apparent.

Since the definition of stress hinges on perception, the investigator needs to rely on self-reporting of the subject relative to their appraisal and perception of stress which deal with psychological and social variables. This raises a problem of verification common to all such endeavors. However, verification by the investigator of the perception of the respondent may not be appropriate or possible. It is a problem that needs to be recognized and accepted as inherent in psychosocial stress research.

Lazarus has also emphasized the transaction nature of stress and that directly implies process, and process implies flux or change. The element of time is thereby introduced into the measurement of stress. Perhaps measurements should be taken over time or at intervals appropriate to some psychosocial situations. The usual psychometric testing currently employed by many investigators tends to measure the instantaneous responses of individuals rather than the many responses of a single individual over time. The reality of field research is that the instantaneous normative approach is usually more easily completed by the investigator than is the ipsative approach which tends to be more longitudinal. Validity may be increased by sampling at various intervals of time since measurement may more closely parallel the transaction process. If one is left with momentary glimpses of the process, one must realize that only part of the stress transaction may be ascertained.

The problem for "those who adopt this emphasis is the difficulty of developing research methods suitable to flux and change as opposed to stability" (Lazarus, 1978,

p. 15). The instruments frequently utilized to measure stress tend to freeze the respondent at one point in time and assume that the moment is representative of the respondent's condition at other times. The theoretical case may be argued that in a dynamic state, the appearance of stability is illusory. For instance, a metaphor can be drawn to the photographic representation of the ballet. Though a single snapshot may accurately portray the position of the dancers at a given moment, one would need to see a movie or series of snapshots taken in sequence in order to appreciate the character of the dance as a whole. Too frequently in psychosocial research on stress one is given merely a single snapshot when one needs to see the entire film in order to discern the relationship of the respondents to the variables in question.

In summary the term stress has been defined as the transactional event in which the perceived external or internal demands on an individual tax his or her physiological, psychological, or social resources. The measurement of such events is tempered by the limitations of verifying perceptions, sampling group vs. individual differences, and taking measurements at a given instant in time rather than over the whole time period of the event.

It is with this background in mind that the term stress is used in the discussion of R.N. baccalaureate student stress. The focus of discussion of theoretical frameworks now turns to the second major area: role stress and role strain, for the stress described in the literature evolves as the R.N. students change roles from technical to professional nurses.

Role Stress and Role Strain: R.N. Socialization

Socialization is defined by Hurley (1978) as the process which prepares "individuals with the general knowledge, skills, and dispositions that will enable them to function as able members of their societies" (p. 65). In the symbolic interaction perspective of socialization favored by Turner (1962), attention is focused on the meaning which "the acts and symbols of actors in the process of interaction have for each other" (Conway, 1978, p. 20). In this context, role is defined by Hardy (1978) as the "expected and the actual behaviors associated with a position" held by the actors or role occupants (p. 75). Hardy (1978) further defines role stress as a problematic social condition which leads to an individual internal response (strain).

Hardy postulates that prevailing social conditions such as inadequate adult socialization, rapid changes in social organization, and accelerated technology all contribute to the role stress and strain seen today (1978, p. 79). Altogether, six types of role problems are identified by Hardy (1978): role ambiguity, role conflict, role incongruity, role overload, role incompetence and role overqualification. Each may be part of role stress which in turn creates role strain.

Overqualification and incompetence refer to the excess resources or deficit of resources that a role occupant holds for a given position. Overload occurs when the role occupant is capable but pressed by excessive demands such as time which prevent fulfilling role obligations. Role conflict exists when existing role expectations are contradictory or mutually exclusive. Role ambiguity may occur when the expectations for a given role are lacking in clarity, vague, or ill-defined.

But the sixth and final type of role stress is of greatest interest: role incongruity.

Hardy defines role incongruity as an instance where "a role occupant finds that expectations for his role performance run counter to his self-perception, disposition, attitudes and values" (1978, p. 82). Hardy further notes that "socialization into one of the professions" can "create conflict between the individual's values and those of the profession" (p. 82). This incongruity is a specific type of role stress then that can occur in professional transitions.

Goode (1960) has provided a definition of role strain, the inevitable consequence of role stress, as the felt difficulty in fulfilling role obligations, a subjective response to role problems. In relating these concepts of socialization to Lazarus' concepts of stress, certain commonalities emerge: the emphasis on the transactional nature of the process, the quality of perception as seen in cognitive appraisal and symbolic interaction, the implied exceeding of resources and the implied interaction between social and psychological systems.

However, consideration of the R.N. baccalaureate student focuses attention on a very specific role which constitutes the third theoretical area under discussion: the characteristics of the adult learner.

The Dreyfus Model of Skill Acquisition

Dreyfus and Dreyfus (1980) have developed a model which describes the stages through which adult learners acquire specific skills. This work was based on the observation of pilots in training and chess players. The model postulates that in the acquisition and eventual mastery of a skill, the learner passes through five levels of development. These separate levels reflect a change in mental capacities dependent on the learner's previous experience. This model was first introduced into nursing by Benner (1980, 1982) and has been used by her to examine the movement of nurses from novice to expert in the work setting.

The model identifies four parts to the mental process giving rise to five levels of performance (Dreyfus, 1981). This is summarized in the chart presented in Table 2 (Dreyfus, 1981, p. 25). As the learner moves up the performance ladder, new capacities are mastered. Each capacity will be examined briefly.

TABLE 2

The Dreyfus Model of Skill Acquisition

Mental Capacity \ Skill Level	NOVICE	ADVANCED BEGINNER	COMPETENT	PROFICIENT	EXPERT
Component Recognition	Nonsituational	Situational	Situational	Situational	Situational
Salience Recognition	None	None	Present	Present	Present
Whole Situation Recognition	Analytical	Analytical	Analytical	Holistic	Holistic
Decision	Rational	Rational	Rational	Rational	Intuitive

Adapted from Dreyfus, S., 1981

In the initial stages, the novice learner has no previous life experience with a given situation. The novice must rely entirely on verbally explicit, context-free rules that govern the behavior in question. As an example, Benner (1982) has cited the example of a context-free rule for dealing with a patient's fluid balance. The novice might be instructed to check daily weights, chart input and output, and if weight gain plus net intake exceeds 500 cc., then place patient on fluid restriction. The instruction can be transmitted totally in the abstract, away from the bedside, and the novice learner would have a reasonable idea of how to proceed without any prior experience. The instruction is not specific to any given patient or any specific situation.

At the next level, advanced beginner, the learner is experiencing a situation for the first few times. Typically the instructor will begin to point out what Dreyfus refers to as recurrent meaningful components or aspects. The instructor can formulate or the learner can develop guidelines which help analyze the situation into meaningful components, but all aspects are equally important. The advanced beginner may recognize the aspects of the situation but is unable to relate them in order of relative importance. Benner (1982) makes this clear in a quote from an expert clinician who was instructing beginning nurses in a pediatric intensive care setting:

If I say, you have to do these eight things, they do those things. They don't stop if another baby is screaming its head off. When they do realize that the other child needs attention, they're like mules between two piles of hay (p. 404).

In Table 1 this ability to discriminate between relative importance of aspects is termed salience recognition. This capacity to think of aspects of a situation in terms of long-range goals or a consciously selected plan is characteristic of the next level up the performance ladder: the competent learner.

The learner at the competent level has had many repetitive exposures to the situation at hand, can readily identify and prioritize the aspects of the situation at hand, and plan her behavior with some level of efficiency and organization to accomplish stated goals. Rather than simply reacting to a barrage of stimuli and demands with equally reflexive responses, the competent performer can pick and choose those behaviors which will maximize the goal.

The next level of performance however represents a quantum leap in capacities. The proficient performer has encountered the situation in many similar circumstances. As Benner notes:

Whereas the competent person does not yet have enough experience to recognize a situation in terms of an overall picture or in terms of which aspects are most salient and most important, the proficient performer now considers fewer options and hones in on an accurate region of the problem. Aspects stand out to the proficient nurse as being more or less important to the situation at hand (p. 405).

This ability to see the situation holistically or from a whole perspective, allows the learner to recognize what is missing as well as what is present. By experiencing the current situation as similar to previous brain-stored, experience-created scenarios, the proficient learner sees the situation through a perspective that is almost anticipatory.

The proficient learner can be guided by what Dreyfus (1981) refers to as maxims, verbal statements meant to convey subtle nuances of a situation that are meaningful only to learners who have a deep understanding of the situation. The experienced surgical nurse who assesses a post-operative patient and warns an equally experienced colleague that the patient "looks sour", or the oncologic nurse who informs the physician that a dying patient has "turned his face to the wall" are communicating their deep understanding of the current situations based on many similar previous encounters. These subtle judgments escape the notice of performers at lower levels. But the proficient learner has mastered the material enough to move from the analytical ordered components recognized by the competent learner to a view of the situation as a whole.

The expert performer no longer relies solely on analytical principle to provide understanding of a situation. Dreyfus (1982) points out:

> Now his repertoire of experienced situations is so vast that normally each specific unresolved situation seen with particular saliences due to prior experience and recent history immediately dictates an intuitively appropriate response. This intuition is possible because each typical whole salienced situation, unconsciously synthesized from several experienced concrete situations..., now has associated with it a specific response or type of response which experience has shown to be appropriate (p. 22).

Benner (1982) recognizes the difficulties in trying to describe performance at the expert level because it is difficult to capture the process in verbal parameters. As an example, she quotes an expert psychiatric nurse:

> When I say to a doctor, "The patient is psychotic," I don't always know how to legitimize that statement. But I am never wrong because I know psychosis from the inside out. And I feel that, and I know it, and I trust it (p.406).

It should be emphasized that if the expert is frustrated or mistaken by an inappropriate choice, she can fall back to lower level analytic processes to solve the problem. But it appears that for the most part, the expert relies on repeated pattern recognition in a nonverbal, nonanalytical way to match appropriate choice of behavior to vast similar past experiences.

In summary, in the Dreyfus Model, the adult learner moves from abstract context-free rules through experiential learning with aspects, salience recognition, holistic perspective and finally expert performance on an experienced, intuitive level. The model is highly dependent on learner perception, is transactional or process oriented, may be equivalent to several levels of learning roles. Utilizing the concepts of Hardy (1978) and Goode (1960), the various levels of performance defined by Dreyfus may be viewed in the socialization context as roles with unique abilities, expectancies, and obligations. While the model addressed uni-directional movement up the performance scale, Benner (1980) has hinted that downward movement can occur when someone operating at a higher level is expected to perform at a lower level.

Benner has observed that if a learner is already functioning at the competent level, recognizing aspects and saliency and selecting behaviors based on long-term goals and plans, the learner may have difficulty when asked to cite the context-free rules and aspects that she no longer depends on for problem-solving. Benner claims that two things occur: 1) the student loses confidence since the rules cannot be as readily cited as when passing through the novice stage, and 2) the instructor can readily lose credibility since it is a simple matter for the experienced competent learner to point out many examples of exceptions to the context-free rules. Benner (1980) states:

> To provide proficient performers with context-free principles and rules will leave them somewhat frustrated and will usually stimulate the experienced nurse to provide examples of situations where clearly the principle or rule would be contradicted. At this point proficient performers can come to feel that theory is a useless trapping. Or they may view the educator's elaborate decision analysis as the hard and unnecessarily elaborate, slow way to solve a clinical problem that they can grasp quickly by virtue of their experience (p. 10).

Dreyfus (1980) has found some empirical data to support this observation. During his study of Air Force pilots in training, Dreyfus noted several phenomena. The instructors could scan the airplane instrument panels much more rapidly and consistently identify problems earlier than the students. The student pilots were given very specific instructions by the instructors on the manner and order in which to visually scan the instrument panels. However, when the eye movements of the instructors were actually measured, the Air Force researchers found that the instructors did not follow the guidelines they had elaborated but in fact scanned the panel in changing patterns appropriate to a given situation. By adapting their pattern unconsciously to the given situations, they more rapidly identified the early errors shown by the instruments. When the instructors were forced to follow the prescribed guidelines for scanning the instrument panels, their efficiency and accuracy in detecting the errors rapidly deteriorated.

This would suggest that to a certain extent each level of performance may correspond to a role (a prescribed set of behaviors) and that movement can proceed from higher role to lower role as well as the expected progression from lower role to higher role. How then can the three major areas of concern (stress, role strain and adult learning) be reconciled to give insight into the position of the R.N. student returning to school for the baccalaureate degree?

Implications for Research

Consideration of these theoretical areas gives rise to several speculations concerning the R.N. baccalaureate student. There is no question that the profession views these students as people who are leaving one role behind to assume a new role, moving from technical to professional nurse (ANA, 1978). There is considerable evidence that suggests these students feel a sense of conflict about this role transition (Hillsmith, 1978; Woolley, 1978; Muzio, 1979; Wilson, 1979). There is evidence to suggest that a discrepancy exists between the way the professional educators perceive these students (Woolley, 1978) and the way the students view their own level of performance (Hillsmith, 1978).

This satisfies the concepts set forth by Hardy (1978) and Goode (1960) for role stress, specifically role incongruity (Hardy, 1978). What may further add to this role stress (conflict between perception of roles) is the impact of the baccalaureate curriculum on these students. Certainly the generic curriculum is typically aimed at the novice learner, a person with no prior experience. Yet particularly with regard to technical skills and perhaps with regard to some professional skills, many R.N. students perceive themselves as functioning at a level above novice, at least advanced beginner, and probably even competent in some cases.

Regardless of the form of the curriculum, if the R.N. student who perceives herself as functioning at a higher level (a higher role) is expected to perform for the sake of the curriculum at a lower level (assume a lower role) one might anticipate an aggravation of already existing role stress and a further impediment to learning. Increased role stress leads to higher role strain, perceived as internal anxiety, tension, frustration, and failure to advance in learning. This may account for the increased attrition, frustration, and personal turmoil documented in these students (Wilson, 1978).

Consideration of these issues may pose a number of questions to be addressed by investigators. The relationship between perception, stress, performance levels, and curricula may be established by examination of their component parts. These relationships may be more simply elucidated by the following questions:

1) What is the self-perception of the R.N. student with regard to performance levels on professional and technical issues at the time of entry into the baccalaureate programs?

2) Does this perception differ significantly from those of other generic students? From associate degree students? From students enrolling in other academic programs?

3) Does a higher level of performance (self-described) in R.N. students correlate with a higher level of role stress and role strain when compared with other R.N. students with lower levels of performance? When compared with other generic students?

4) Are there differences in levels of role stress and role strain encountered by R.N. students who are involved in degree programs in different settings or different degree programs, e.g., second-step programs vs. generic programs?

5) Does role stress and role strain in R.N. students interfere with personal growth and learning?

Addressing these questions would aid in the development of programs which would facilitate the movement of R.N. students into and through the baccalaureate programs. Nursing would benefit, the R.N. student would benefit, and the patients would ultimately benefit from higher level, professional care.

REFERENCES

American Nurses' Association. *Facts about nursing 80-81*. New York: American Journal of Nursing, 1981.

American Nurses' Association. News. *American Journal of Nursing*, 1982, *82*(4), 518-520.

American Nurses' Association. Resolutions. *The American Nurse*, 1978, *10*(9), 9-10.

Badossi, K. In search of the BSN ... programs for practicing RNs. Why BSN programs drive nurses crazy. *RN*, 1980, *43*, 52-55.

STRESS OF THE RETURNING R.N. STUDENT

Balogh, E. RN students analyze their experiences. *Nursing Outlook*, 1970, *28*, 112-115.

Banertscher, B. Obstacle course on professional education. *Arizona Nurse*, 1979, *32*, 6.

Benner, P. Characteristics of novice and expert performance: Implications for teaching the experienced nurse. Paper presented at "Researching Second Step Nursing Education," January 12-13, 1980, San Francisco, California.

Benner, P. From novice to expert. *American Journal of Nursing*, 1982, *82*, 402-407.

Boddie, B. Diploma grad tells why she supports BSN for entry. *American Nurse*, 1970, *12*, 4-5.

Brown, J.S., Swift, Y.B., & Oberman, M.L. Baccalaureate students' images of nursing: A replication. *Nursing Research*, 197, *23*, 53-59.

Choinski, C. Playing with the entry requirement: A game we can't afford . . . what nursing is in 1978 and what it will be in 1985. *RN*, 1978, *41*, 27-28.

Conway, M. Theoretical approaches to the study of roles. In M. Hardy and M. Conway (Eds.), *Role theory: Perspectives for health professionals*. New York: Appleton-Century-Crofts, 1978.

de Tornyay, R. Proposed changes in academic preparation for nursing practice: Implications for the health care system and the educational system. In *Changes in nursing education: Implications for practice* (79-Serial No. 1). Washington, D.C.: American Association of Colleges of Nursing, 1979.

Diploma schools fight ANA proposal. *Modern Health Care*, 1980, *10*, 46.

Dreyfus, S. *Formal models vs. human situational understanding: Inherent limitations on the modeling of business expertise*. Berkeley: University of California, 1981.

Dreyfus, S., & Dreyfus, H. *A five-stage model of the mental activities involved in direct skill acquisition*. Berkeley: University of California, 1980.

Galliford, S. Second step baccalaureate programs in nursing. *Nursing Outlook*, 1978, *26*, 98-102.

Glass, D., & Esch, C.J. Professionalization of Nursing Students in Second Step Programs. In K. Jako (Ed.), *Researching Second Step Nursing Education*. Vol. 2. Rohnert Park, CA: Sonoma State University, 1981.

Goode, W. A theory of role strain. *American Sociological Review*, 1960, *25*, 483-496.

Gortner, S.R. Nursing Majors in Twelve Western Universities: A Comparison of Registered Nurse Students and Basic Senior Students. *Nursing Research*, 1968, *17*, 121-128.

Hardy, M. Role stress and role strain. In M. Hardy and M. Conway (Eds.), *Role theory: Perspectives for health professionals*. New York: Appleton-Century-Crofts, 1978.

Hillsmith, K. From RN to BSN: Student perceptions. *Nursing Outlook*, 1978, *26*, 631-635.

Kidd, J. *How adults learn.* New York: Association Press, 1977.

La Violette, S. Hospital associations oppose 1985 proposal...that all professional nurses have baccalaureate degrees after 1982. *Hospital Progress,* 1979, *9,* 44-45.

Lazarus, R. The stress and coping paradigm. Paper presented at a conference entitled "The critical evaluation of behavioral paradigms for psychiatric science," Gelenden Beach, Oregon, November 1978, 1-52.

Lazarus, R., Cohen, J., et al. Psychological stress and adaptation: Some unresolved issues. In H. Selye (Ed.), *Selye's guide to stress research* (vol. 1). New York: Van Nostrand Reinhold, 1980, 90-117.

Lazarus, R., & Launier, R. Stress-related transactions between person and environment. In L.A. Pervin and M. Lewis (Eds.), *Perspectives in interactional psychology.* New York: Plenum Press, 1978, 287-327.

McGettigan, B. Non-nursing degree for RNs examined. *California Nurse,* 1970, *75,* 9.

McKay, S. A review of student stress in nursing education programs. *Nursing Forum,* 1978, *17,* 376-393.

Macmasters, E. Sources of stress in university nursing students. *Nursing Papers,* 1979, *11,* 87-96.

Mallory, S.L. A Comparison of Registered Nurse Students in Generic and Second Step Baccalaureate Programs, (Doctoral Dissertation, Kansas State University, Makihattan, Kansas 1982).

Maslow, A. *The farther reaches of human nature.* New York: Viking Press, 1971.

Mason, J. A historical view of the stress field. *Journal of Human Stress,* 1975, *2,* 22.

Meyer, G.R., *Tenderness and Technique: Nursing Values in Transition,* Los Angeles: Institute of Industrial Relations, 1960.

Mullendore, T.L. "Interrelationships of Self-Esteem, Internal-External Locus of Control, Age, Marital Status and Grade Point Average among the Registered Nurse Students in a Baccalaureate Program," (Unpublished Master's Thesis, 1974), cited in Gray, F.S. Socialization of the R.N. in baccalaureate nursing education. In *Baccalaureate Nursing Education for Registered Nurses: Issues and Approaches,* (Published November 15-18[12]). New York: National League for Nursing, 1980.

Muzio, L., & Ohashi, J. The RN student — unique characteristics, unique needs. *Nursing Outlook,* 1979, *27,* 528-532.

National League for Nursing. *State-approved schools of nursing, R.N. 1980.* NLN pub. no. 19-1823. New York: Author, 1980.

Nyquist, E. The external degree program and nursing. *Nursing Outlook,* 1973, *21,* 372-377.

STRESS OF THE RETURNING R.N. STUDENT

Rosenstein, A. Future of education for the profession. *Education Digest,* 1978, *44,* 2-6.

Selye, H. *Stress without distress.* Philadelphia: Lippincott, 1974.

Shane, D. The returning-to-school syndrome. *Nursing 80, 10,* 86-90.

Styles, M. *On nursing: Toward a new endowment.* St. Louis: C.V. Mosby, 1982.

Tourneau, L. Want a BSN? Try and get it. *RN,* 1970, *43,* 75-76.

Turner, R. Role-taking: Process versus conformity. In A. Rose (Ed.), *Human behavior and social process. An interactionist approach.* Boston: Houghton Mifflin, 1962.

Vaillant, G. *Adaptation to life.* Boston: Little, Brown & Co., 1977.

Wilson, H. Why RN students dropout. *Nursing Outlook,* 1978, *26,* 437-441.

Woolley, A. From RN to BSN: Faculty perceptions. *Nursing Outlook,* 1978, *26,* 103-108.

Zorn, J. A research profile of today's baccalaureate nursing student. *Journal of Continuing Education in Nursing,* 1980, *11,* 7-9.

PART TWO:
NURSING EDUCATION
IN THE SERVICE SETTING

Chapter Six:
Stress and Critical Care Nursing

Chapter Six:
Stress and Critical Care Nursing

June T. Bailey, R.N., Ed.D., F.A.A.N.
Lillian A. Bargagliotti, R.N., M.S.

Investigative studies of psychologic stress of hospital nurses, particularly job-related stress of Critical Care Nurses,[1] reflect a heightened interest among researchers. A computerized literature search indicates that some one hundred articles on stress of nurses have been published during the past two decades. An initial review of these articles reported in the 1960's, 70's and 80's suggests that the majority of studies centered on stress of Intensive Care and/or Coronary Care Nurses. One of the reasons for the ever-increasing interest of researchers in studying stress of nurses in these highly specialized units may well be that these units represent a relatively new and innovative approach to health care delivery, having originated in the 60's. New knowledge and technical advances in complex medical and surgical procedures such as heart and kidney transplantations, coronary-artery-by pass surgery, and other complex interventions have signaled the need for an expanded role of the nurse. The new and expanded role of the Critical Care Nurse is characterized by increased autonomy, responsibility, and for accountability in maintaining high standards of performance. In addition, these specialty units represent a drama of living and dying among the critically ill in a fast-paced environment. For example, the Critical Care Nurse is surrounded by an array of complex machinery and is required to maintain a constant vigilence of flashing monitors and to note momentary changes in the patient's condition. Moreover, responding to a "Code-Blue" and initiating life-saving measures, as well as dealing with death and dying on a daily basis become a vital part of the care giving role. These phenomena which encompass new roles and new settings herald a need for synthesizing and summarizing major findings of studies of psychologic stress of Critical Care Nurses, and to chart new directions for future research on stress.

Significance of Stress of Critical Care Nurses

The stress of nurses in Critical Care Units achieves significance as a problem because of the inherent potential for adversely affecting the quality of patient care as well as the health and well-being of the nurse. However, empirical data concerning the effect of stress upon the health of the nurse and/or the quality of patient care have not been reported to date. The relationship between the stress of nurses and its effect on patient care has primarily been broached from the perspectives of the nursing shortage or the high attrition rate among nurses. Millar (1980, p. 802) contends that frustration and dissatisfaction with work leads to nurses "voting with their feet." Wandelt (1981) also supports the notion that nurses are leaving their profession. In contrast to the position taken by Millar and Wandelt relative to nurses leaving their positions, Aiken (1981) contends that 75% of all nurses

---

[1]Throughout the chapter, Critical Care Nurses refers to nurses working on Intensive Care Units, Coronary Care Units, or Neonatal Intensive Care Units.

licensed in the United States are employed in nursing, giving nursing the distinction of having one of the highest rates of labor participation of any female dominated occupation. Furthermore the finding that only 4.1% of nurses are employed in non-nursing fields casts further doubt on the notion of a "flight from nursing" (*Facts About Nursing,* 1981). Of the 25% of the nurse population who are inactive, the American Nurses' Association reports that the majority of nurses are over the age of 50. The majority of nurses who are under the age of 40 have young children at home (*Facts About Nursing,* 1981). However positive this data appears, it is overshadowed by the American Nurses' Association's (1981) finding that only 52% of employed nurses are practicing on a full-time basis. Part-time practice is of concern because of the following trends: (1) higher acuity level of hospitalized patients; (2) extended ages of the population; and (3) the increased incidence of chronic disease in the United States. These factors portend an added demand for nursing services.

In addition to the concern that nurses are leaving nursing, the rate of job-turnover has captured the attention of nursing administrators. The data on job-turnover of nurses is somewhat questionable since hospitals actively engaged in recruitment appear to be reluctant to accurately publicize turnover rates of their nurses. The American Nurses' Association reports a job-turnover rate for the entire nurse population of 40%, and the National Association of Nurse Recruiters cite a national rate of 32% (Wolfe, 1981). A national survey of 1,111 Directors of Nursing was conducted to determine why Intensive Care or Coronary Care Nurses in their particular institution were leaving nursing (Robinson, 1972). The results of the survey indicated the following: (1) 43% of Critical Care Nurses resigned because of pregnancy; (2) 49% left because of relocation; and, (3) 8% left for stated reasons of "fatigue and pressure" (Robinson, 1972, p. 47). The reliability of this data may raise some questions since the respondents were Directors of Nursing. However, Grout, Steffen, and Bailey's (1980) regional study of Intensive Care Nurses (n = 1238) lends support to these findings. Of the 58% of their nursing sample who had worked in other critical care settings, over half of the CCU nurses listed personal reasons for leaving. The most frequent response given was that the nurse had moved. Approximately 2% of the sample listed work related stress as a cause for having left a Critical Care Unit. A relevant question arises as to whether or not pregnancy and relocation represent a more acceptable reason for resigning rather than to admit to a difficult work situation. Although conclusive data are lacking for turnover rates and causative factors, Donovan's (1980) national survey of 223 hospitals indicated that 90% of Directors of Nursing reported full-time nursing vacancies which they were unable to fill. In addition, 51% of the Directors of Nursing considered the shortage to be most acute in critical care areas.

A discussion of job-turnover and the discrepencies noted indicate that conclusions from statistics on job-turnover must be viewed with caution as nursing is one of the professions in which monopsony occurs (Aiken, 1981). Nurses may be stressed and dissatisfied; however, they may remain in their jobs because of a realistic or preceived lack of options.

Criteria and Rationale for Selected
Studies on Stress of Critical Care Nurses

CRITERIA Since an inordinate number of *studies* on stressors of CCU nurses (some 30 investigations) have been reported in the literature and reviewed by the authors, it became apparent that criteria need to be developed in order to select a reasonable number of studies to be evaluated. The following criterion measures were developed and applied: (1) studies selected for review should focus primarily on the variable of identifying psychologic stressors of nurses employed on units designated as Intensive Care, Coronary Care, or Neonatal Intensive Care units in hospitals in this country; (2) the design, analysis, and findings should be reported; (3) comparative studies of stressors of CCU nurses with nurses employed on other units will *not* be included; and (4) of the studies which met criterion measures one, two, and three, further selection should include a sample of Studies of Stress of Critical Care Nurses published in 1960, 1970, and 1980.

RATIONALE FOR SELECTION PROCESS The rationale for the stated criteria in the selection of seven studies to be reviewed in this chapter is primarily threefold: (1) baseline data on the perceived, psychologic *stressors* of Critical Care Nurses are requisite if further investigations on stress of nurses are to proceed; (2) although the stressors of approximately 1800 intensive care nurses have been identified and reported by one of the authors, (JTB), the next step appeared to be to examine the extent to which the finding relative to identified stressors in the Bailey, et al. studies (1980) is congruent with studies conducted by other investigators whose primary purpose was to identify and/or rank the stressors. It would appear that if there were commonalities in the findings, irrespective of the investigator, the design, or analysis, that investigator bias might be negated and that the implication for nursing education and nursing service might be strengthened; and, (3) the decision to select studies of Stress of CCU Nurses from a sample of studies conducted during the 60's, 70's and 80's was made in order to determine from a historical perspective whether or not there appeared to be trends in methodology or similarities in findings.

Theoretical Framework for Stress

THE STRESS PARADIGMS The stress paradigm encompasses primarily two major schools of thought. Selye, the "Father of the stress concept," has studied the nature of stress for fifty years and has presented a biological-physiological model. He defines stress as "the nonspecific response of the body to any demand made upon it." (Selye, 1975, p. 38). The nonspecific physiologic response proposed by Selye is known as the General Adaptation Syndrome which is comprised of three phases: (1) the alarm phase, (2) the resistance phase, and, (3) the exhaustion phase. During the alarm phase, physiologic changes occur which can be quantified through procedures which purport to measure physiologic stress. For example, there is an increased outflow of catecholamines from the adrenal medulla which results in increased heart rate, increased blood pressure, and enhancement of clotting. A concomitant increased outflow of corticoids from the adrenal cortex results in multiple changes such as gluconeogenesis and the inhibition of inflammatory response (Selye, 1980, p. 129). The phase of resistance occurs if successful adaptation has been possible and physical signs of the alarm phase disappear. When the stressor continues and resistance cannot be maintained, the phase of exhaustion occurs and signs of the alarm phase reappear. During this phase, Selye (1980) argues that the signs of the alarm phase are now irreversible and inadequate and as a consequence the individual dies. Selye also postulated that the energy available for adaptation to stressors is finite, thus suggesting that control of stress is necessary for survival. Furthermore, Selye contends that one can control the response to a stressor by determining which situations are worthy of response.

Lazarus proposes a psychosocial stress model and defines stress as "any event in which environmental or internal demand (or both) tax or exceed the adaptive resources of an individual (Lazarus, 1981, p. 192). Lazarus maintains that it is one's "cognitive appraisal" of the stressor that determines one's response to it. A basic assumption of Lazarus' theory of stress, which has both principled and constructive beginnings, is that stress is neither a stimulus nor a response but that stress arises from the transaction between the demand or environment stimulus and the person's perception and cognitive appraisal of the situation. The transaction is appraised as irrelevant, benign/positive, or stressful. If the situational demand is perceived as stressful, further appraisal by the individual determines whether the situation is one which represents harm/loss, threat, or challenge. Cognitive appraisal considers the degree of threat, location of the stressor, and the availability of viable options. In considering differences in vulnerability to stress, it has been suggested by Lazarus that the situation must be of a given intensity and of a given kind to produce stress in a particular person. Consequently, predictions of stress of an individual arise from a knowledge of conditioning factors such as heredity, educational experiences, values, goals, and life experiences.

Lazarus' recent approach (1981) to the study of stress is reported in a preliminary study (n = 100) of daily "Hassles" and "Uplifts." The investigation was based on the premise that it is the minor, daily, irritating, frustrating events or hassles, such as losing something, that prove to be better predictors of stress, providing the hassles are not counterbalanced with uplifts or challenges. Factors considered to be uplifts were identified, but did not appear to buffer the effects of hassles (Lazarus, 1981). Although numerous scales of Lazarus' instrument are available, further empirical investigation is needed.

DISCUSSION OF THE STRESS PARADIGMS Stress as a paradigm, while enjoying numerous discussions in the literature, evokes a number of theoretical problems. The lack of precision in defining the conceptual boundaries of the stress concept has resulted in its use as a stimulus, response, or intervening construct (Eisdorfer, 1981; Mason, 1975). An additional limitation to theoretical development and empirical investigation has been the reductionistic, fragmented approach to stress as either a biological, psychological, or sociological phenomena. (Lazarus, 1981; Mason, 1975; Eisdorfer, 1981). Theoretical linkages between and among biological, psychological, and sociological man are notably absent, creating a theoretical gap. Mason (1975) attempted to bridge the gap by suggesting that psychologic arousal (cognitive appraisal) might well be the elusive first mediator sought by Selye. However, Selye (1975) refuted this notion by citing the occurrence of the physiological stress response in plants, lower animals, and anesthetized unconscious patients where neurological systems were absent or non-functioning. The conceptual schism remains. Lazarus (1981) is beginning to cite the need for empirical investigations of stress at the biological, psychological, and sociological levels, whereas Eisdorfer (1981) and Pelletier (1977) advocate an holistic theoretical approach. However, holistic measures of stress await development. Levels of physiological stress can only be inferred from the use of comparative data (Melton et al., 1973; Polis et al., 1969).

The two contrasting empirical approaches to stress, Selye's laboratory approach (1975) and Lazarus' naturalistic, ipsative-normative approach (1981), reflect the range of controversy concerning reliability. Regardless of setting or conceptual framework, the measures on stress continue to be problematic because of intra-subject variability that is unrelated to the presence of stressors (Garbin, 1979). The feasibility of using physiological measures remains problematic because of the availability of subjects, the intrusive nature of the process, and the high cost of laboratory procedures. The current state of divergent approaches with conflicting strengths and weaknesses coupled with problems in design and instrumentation reflect an evolutionary stage of development of the stress paradigms.

Review of Selected Studies on Psychologic Stress of CCU Nurses

Seven studies which met the criterion measures presented earlier will be reviewed relative to the psychologic stress of CCU Nurses. The studies will be organized from an historical approach with a review of selected studies reported in the 1960's, 1970's and 1980's. The methodology and major findings of each of the seven studies are presented in Table 1.

TABLE 1
Summary of Seven Selected Studies of Stress of Clinical Care Nurses

INVESTIGATOR	DESIGN	SAMPLE	METHOD/INSTRUMENTS	FINDINGS (STRESSORS)
Koumans (1965)	Case Study	Four Cases	Participant-Observation	Rapid turnover of staff and patients. Confused, demanding, and/or dying patients. Interpersonal relations between nurse-nurse; nurse-physician; and nurse-patient.
Vreeland and Ellis (1969)	Case Study	ICU Nurses, (N=unreported)	Observation	Patient's condition Knowledge and skill required Urgency of situation requiring constant vigilance Painfulness of nursing measures Level of responsibility Interpersonal relationships
Cassem and Hackett (1972)	Descriptive	CCU Nurses (N=16) Sample of convenience	Questionnaire Forced choice comparison between 7 areas of potential conflict	Heavy lifting Unpredictable staffing/scheduling Overwrought, anxious families Responsibilities Lack of time off Severity of patient's prognosis
Jacobson (1978)	Descriptive	NICU Nurses (N=87) Sample of convenience	Questionnaire of representative incidents identified from 220 anecdotes originally reported as stressful by the sample	Philosophical-emotional problems Nurse-doctor problems Understaffing and overwork Nurse-nurse problems Sudden death or relapse of infant

Table 1 (cont'd)

INVESTIGATOR	DESIGN	SAMPLE	METHOD/INSTRUMENTS	FINDINGS (STRESSORS)
Huckabay and Jagla (1979)	Descriptive	ICU Nurses (N=46) Sample of convenience	Demographic Questionnaire Questionnaire on stressors extracted from selected literature	Work load and amount of physical load Death of a patient Communication problems with staff and nursing office Meeting the needs of the family Communication between staff and physicians
Bailey (1980)	Descriptive	ICU Nurses (N=1794) Sample of convenience	Demographic data Questionnaire (Free Response) on satisfiers/stressors Perceived stressor inventory (PSI)	*Stressors:* (Categories) Management of unit Interpersonal conflict Nature of direct patient care *Satisfiers:* Interpersonal relationships Direct patient care Acquisition of knowledge and skills
Anderson & Basteyns (1981)	Descriptive	ICU Nurses (N=182) Sample of convenience	Questionnaire listing stressors obtained from literature review utilizing Bilodeau's criteria	Death of a young adult Unable to get help when short of staff Physician not available when an emergency arises Making a medication error

SELECTED STUDIES ON PSYCHOLOGIC STRESS OF CRITICAL CARE NURSES (1960's) The *Koumans Study* (1965) identified stressors of Intensive Care Nurses from the perspective of the ICU setting as a community or social unit. Utilizing a participant-observer approach, as presented in Table 1, Koumans, a psychiatrist, met weekly with the nursing staff and participated in biweekly medical rounds on the Intensive Care Units of Massachusetts General Hospital. Based upon observations over a one-year period, three major stressors or "crisis provoking" factors in the intensive care unit were identified: (1) rapid turnover of staff and patients (2) confused, demanding, or dying patients and (3) the "intensity affect" in interpersonal relations between nurse-nurse, nurse-physician, and nurse-patient. Although the limitations of Koumans' case study are numerous, Koumans' qualitative and inductive approach to a relatively new area of research is noteworthy. Pragmatically, findings of the Koumans' study lack external validity due to the small sample size (4 cases). In addition, the sample may well have been one of convenience. Internal validity of the study is limited by the subjectivity of the design.

The *Vreeland and Ellis Study* (1969) identified the stressors of Intensive Care Nurses through observation of nurses at the National Institute of Health, Bethesda, Maryland. Findings of the study indicated that factors related to patient care and interpersonal relations were the most significant stressors of ICU Nurses. As presented in Table 1, the primary stressors were identified as patients condition, knowledge and skills required, urgency of the situation, painfulness of nursing measures, level of responsibility, and interpersonal relationships.

Methodologically, the subjectivity of the investigators, and the failure to report the details of the observations made such as the number and frequency of observations, jeopardize the external validity.

SELECTED STUDIES ON PSYCHOLOGIC STRESS OF CRITICAL CARE NURSES (1970's) The *Cassem and Hackett Study* represents a small descriptive study (n = 16) to identify stressors of Critical Care Nurses. The study was one of the first studies to use instruments rather than to rely on observations to gather the data. Major stressors presented in Table 1 were identified as heavy lifting, unpredictable staffing, overwrought anxious families, responsibility, lack of time off, and severity of the patient's prognosis. It was noted that the validity and the reliability of the Questionnaire designed by the authors were not reported. Small sample size is another major weakness of the study, which limits the generalizability of the findings.

The Jacobson Study (1978) and the Huckabay and Jagla Study (1979) demonstrate a number of commonalities, although the sample in the Jacobson study (n = 87) consisted of nurses employed in the Neonatal Intensive Care Unit, whereas the Huckabay and Jagla study population (n = 46) was comprised on Intensive Care Nurses. Both studies are descriptive as presented in Table 1. The overall purpose of both studies was concerned not only with identifying stressors but with the rank ordering of the stressors. Instruments consisted of a Questionnaire which was used in each of the studies. Some questions of validity of the Questionnaire are raised since the data on the stressors were obtained through forced-choice. However, reliability measures are reported by both investigators. These studies also used a sample of convenience rather than a random sampling procedure. Although the studies report a rank-ordering of stressors, the method of ranking is somewhat unclear in the Huckabay and Jagla study (1979).

Rank-order of the Jacobson study (1978) relative to the identified stressors of Neonatal Intensive Care Nurses were as follows: philosophical-emotional problems, nurse-doctor problems, understaffing and overworked, nurse-nurse problems, and sudden death or relapse of an infant. There is a striking similarity of stressors identified by Huckabay and Jagla (1979) as presented in Table 1. The stressors and the rank order of the Huckabay and Jagla study were: workload and amount of physical work, death of a patient, communication problems with staff and the nursing office, meeting the heads of the family, and communication between staff and physicians.

SELECTED STUDIES OF PSYCHOLOGIC STRESS OF CRITICAL CARE NURSES (1980's)

The Bailey Study (1980) represents a descriptive study whose primary purposes were to establish a large data base on the stressors and satisfiers of Intensive Care Nurse and to partially test Lazarus' concept relative to the role of perception and cognitive appraisal in identifying stressors. Stressors and satisfiers were identified, categorized, and rank ordered through a free response questionnaire (n = 1794). The categories of stressors and their rank order include the following: (1) Interpersonal Conflicts, (2) Management of the Unit, (3) Nature of Direct Patient Care, (4) Inadequate Knowledge and Skills, (5) Physical Work Environment, (6) Life Events, and (7) Lack of Administrative Rewards. It was interesting to note that almost 85% of the stressors were represented in the first three categories.

The stressors of ICU Nurses were identified from a questionnaire which was circulated to a regional, national sample, and local sample of ICU Nurses. In addition to obtaining data on the "Stressors" of ICU Nurses, data were obtained on the "Satisfiers" or challenges of the job perceived by ICU Nurses. Since the theoretical framework of the study incorporated many of Lazarus' concepts of psychosocial stress, it seemed appropriate to partially test the role of *perception* and *congitive appraisal* through identifying both the stressors and satisfiers of the ICU

Nurses. If indeed Lazarus' contention that stress is neither a stimulus nor a response but is the result of the transaction between the person and the environment and that *perception* and *cognitive* appraisal are requisite to identifying stress, then it follows that one way to partially test these concepts might be through collecting data on both the threatening and challenging aspects of stress (Bailey, 1980, p. 24). For example, if one ICU Nurse were to state that responding to a "Code Blue" was a stressor, and another nurse specified that responding to a "Code Blue" was indeed a challenge or satisfier, it would appear that the individual's perception, cognitive appraisal, and conditioning factors did indeed play a role as indicated earlier in the discussion of Lazarus' stress paradigm. The categories and a rank ordering of sources of greatest satifaction are presented in Table 1.

The Nature of Direct Patient Care was ranked as the number one satisfier and represented 48% of the responses whereas Interpersonal Relationship, and Acquisition of Knowledge and Use of Skills were ranked number two and three and represented 46% of the satisfiers. It is important to note that there are striking similarities between the categories of perceived stressors and satisfiers of 1794 ICU nurses (Bailey, pp. 16-24). Interpersonal Conflicts was identified as the number one category of stress whereas Interpersonal Relationships were perceived as the number three satisfier. Moreover, the Nature of Direct Patient Care represented the number one category in which ICU Nurses derived satisfaction, and paradoxically this same category was rank-ordered number three as a stressor. By the same analysis, the use of Knowledge and Skills were perceived as satisfiers and were rank ordered number two.

The stressors of the Intensive Care Nurses in the Bailey Study (1980, p. 16-17) were: conflict with other health care providers, inadequate staffing patterns, lack of support in dealing with emergencies and death, and inadequate work space.

Confidence in findings of the Bailey Studies (1980) is enhanced by the size and representativeness of the sample (n = 1794). Self-selected sample bias is negated by the response rate of 60% for the regional sample (n = 1238) and 57% for the national sample (n = 566). (Claus and Bailey, 1980; Polit and Hungler, 1978, p. 348). Construct validity of the stress audit tool was enhanced by the convergence of free response items with the 43-item forced-choice questionnaire. (Grout, Steffen and Bailey, 1981; Polit and Hungler, 1978, p. 438). Content validity was obtained through the use of an expert panel whose qualifications were cited. (Claus and Bailey, 1980). Reliability of the tool is suggested by the degree of agreement between samples. Inter-rater reliability for categorization of free response items is reported. (Grout, Steffen, and Bailey, 1981).

Aside from the power of the sample size, a significant strength of the Bailey studies (1980) was the approach to identification of stressors. Utilization of free-response questions avoided the problem of artificial limits on the possible set of stressors and of pre-setting the respondent through a checklist. The method used for analysis of the data through Flanagan's Category Formulation is supported by previous research (Bailey, 1956). An additional finding that is worthy of note was the low percentage of nurses (14.9%) who considered their intensive care practice to be stressful (Grout, Steffen, and Bailey, 1981). A major weakness of the study was the non-randomizing of the sample, and the unreported validity and reliability of the instruments.

The *Anderson and Basteyns Study* (1981) used a research format similar to the earlier Huckabay and Jagla (1979) study. Anderson and Basteyns (1981) investigated the stressors of Intensive Care Unit Nurses (n = 182) from 17 hospitals in the Milwaukee area. From an 84-item questionnaire, they obtained a rank ordering of stressors related to patient care and management of the unit which supported the findings of earlier studies. Generalizability of their findings is limited by sample bias, as well as construct and content validity of their instrument. As noted in Table 1, the major stressors and the rank order included the following: (1) death of a young adult, (2) unable to get help when short of (nursing) staff, (3) physician not available when an emergency arises, and, (4) making a medication error.

Summary of Findings

COMMONALITIES AMONG FINDINGS OF THE SEVEN STUDIES   A review of the seven studies suggested the need to develop a method to compare and synthesize the findings on the identified stressors of Critical Care Nurses. The categories identified in the Bailey Studies (1980) appeared to be one method which would lend itself to further comparative analysis of the data. The stressors identified in the seven studies were distributed among the six categories as presented in Table 2.

TABLE 2:

DISTRIBUTIONS OF CATEGORIES OF STRESS OF CCU NURSES IN SEVEN SELECTED STUDIES.[1]

Study	Categories of Stressors					
	Interpersonal Conflict	Nature of Direct Pt. Care	Knowledge and Skills	Management and the Unit	Physical Work Environment	Administrative Rewards or Problems
Koumans (1965)	X[2]	O[1]	X	X	O	O
Vreeland and Ellis (1969)	X	X	X	O	O	O
Cassem and Hackett (1972)	X	X	O	X	X	X
Jacobson (1978)	X	X	X	X	X	X
Huckabay and Jagla (1979)	X	X	X	O	X	O
Bailey (1980) (1980)	X	X	X	X	X	X
Anderson and Basteyns (1981)	X	X	X	X	O	O

1. Since the Bailey study was the only study that used the Life Events Scale, this category of stress was not included in the Table.

2. "X" denotes stressors identified in above categories.

3. "O" denotes stressors not identified in above categories.

The primary stressors of Critical Care Nurses were in the following categories: Interpersonal Conflict, the Nature of Direct Patient Care, Knowledge and Skills, and Management of the Unit. Considering the differences in design, sample size, instrumentation, and methodological limitations, the findings among the seven studies reviewed is striking.

For example, a profile of the Critical Care Nurse begins to emerge. Specifically, the Critical Care Nurse might well be described as one who is stressed by: (1) conflicts with other health care providers, patients, and their families; (2) the workload and inadequate staffing; and (3) dealing with death and dying, and responding to emergencies.

HISTORICAL PERSPECTIVE ON THE FINDINGS From an historical approach, it is interesting to note that studies presented in the 1960's were essentially case studies using observation. The primary purpose of studies conducted in the 60's was to recognize Critical Care Nursing as stressful. The 1970's reflect increased sophistication in methodology with the use of instruments to collect data but with problems in content validity and in reliability of findings. The 1970's also indicate not only a concern for identifying the stressors but also an analysis of the data to rank order the stressors.

Studies in the 1980's represent a larger sample size (n = 182 and n = 1794) and more detailed analysis of the data. Attention is also given to the context in which critical care nursing is practiced with description of the units and the hospital setting. The 1980's might also be described as a time for reflection and for furthering the advancement of knowledge relevant to stress in nursing.

Limitations on the Studies of Nursing Stress

Inextricably related to stress is the environment or content within which nursing practice occurs. The nature of the critical care unit provides one context for the stressors and satisfiers of nurses. Consideration of context as an independent variable is a notable omission in most of the studies of critical care stressors. Observers have dramatically, and somewhat normatively, described the intensive care unit as a "war bunker" and a place of "pain, delirium, and death" (Hay and Oken, 1972; Cassem and Hackett, 1975; Gentry et al., 1972). For empirical purposes, objective description of the practice setting in terms of nurse-patient ratio, acuity level of patients, average length of patient stay, physical characteristics of the unit, the administration structure, and the relationship of nursing to other disciplines would provide an important perspective for empirical findings and could serve as a basis from which valid generalizations could be made. Bailey et al.'s (1980) study of stressors of critical care nurses (n = 1794) provides one example of the usefulness of considering the context of the situation. For example, findings in the Stanford sample (n = 129) differed in some areas from those of the regional and national samples, reflecting that the Stanford setting which is characterized as a complex, specialized acute care center may have accounted for the fact that Stanford Critical Care Nurses were *significantly* more stressed by the physical work environment than the nurses in the regional or national sample (Bailey, Steffen and Grout, 1980, p. 15). The above finding illustrates that not only is the content of the situation important, but also the work setting. Although the work setting of an acute care hospital has been described from a myriad of perspectives, it has recently been characterized as patriarchal and misogynous (Ashley, 1980). Nursing is noted for having minimal control over the patient care setting, which places the nurse in a position that has been described as "low man on the totem pole" (Lewis, 1976, p. 24; Wolf, 1981). Smith (1972) has conceptualized the hospital as a normative organization that is becoming more utilitarian because of unionization and the concern for cost effectiveness. Normative organizations are those obtaining compliance from subordinates through internalization by the subordinate of organizational norms and values. In contrast, utilitarian organizations obtain compliance from subordinates through the control of material resources and rewards.

Consideration of the context provides a requisite frame of reference for the study of stress in nursing practice. Although nursing occurs in a complex environment, it seems necessary to isolate the salient features of the environment. Such an appraisal identifies a focus for research as well as a number of independent variables which should be considered.

In addition to the lack of attention in most of the studies relative to the context in which Critical Care Nurses practice, the sampling procedures in each of the studies reviewed limit the findings. Most of the studies suffered from small sample size. In addition, none of the studies used a randomized sampling procedure, but reported using samples which were ones of convenience.

A number of other methodological problems were apparent in most of the studies as discussed earlier, such as reliability and validity measures of the instruments, incomplete reporting on the data analysis, and lack of a theoretical framework.

Implications for Nursing Service and Nursing Education

Nursing service and nursing education need to develop increased awareness on the nature and power of stress. The phenomena of stress is inherent not only in the complex nature of nursing education and practice, but it also pervades the lives of each of us. Furthermore, stress and its relationship to health and illness have been well documented, and should be of particular concern to nursing educators and health care providers. As first steps, well developed recruitment and orientation programs for new faculty or nursing service staff need to be expanded: the roles, expectation, and evaluation procedures should be well defined to prevent role conflict or role ambiguity. Stress audits of personnel need to be conducted, analyzed, and appropriate actions need to be taken to deal more effectively with the identified stressors of nurses.

Since the category of *Interpersonal Conflict* was identified in each of the studies reviewed earlier as the category which caused nurses distress and was frequently ranked as the number one stressor, both nursing service and nursing education need to be more concerned with "people problems." Courses and inservice education programs need to be offered in Conflict Management. In addition, lines of communication need to be kept open in both service and educational organizations and the use of feedback needs to be strengthened.

The category on the Nature of Direct Patient Care was identified in four of the studies as a stressor. Dealing with death and dying were particularly stressful. Initiation of courses and programs dealing with these concerns, such as courses on bio-ethics, need to be initiated if they are not already in place.

Management of the Unit was a category which was perceived by a majority of nurses as a source of stress. This finding heralds a call for providing nurses *knowledge* in management and leadership, and a call for action on the part of nursing service directors to provide sufficient and competent staff for critical care units.

Requisite Knowledge and Skills in the nursing care-giving role also needs attention from nursing educators and nursing service directors. Nursing educators should recognize Critical Care Nursing as a highly specialized role within a complex practice setting which requires new knowledge and skills, and adequate preparation. Nursing service directors, supervisors, and/or head nurses should be aware of the need for specialized training in this area of care and either employ nurses who have critical care training or provide programs to increase the knowledge and skill base of CCU Nurses. There is also a need for Nursing Service Administrators to become more familiar with highly specialized Critical Care Units and the inherent stressors of nurses who deal with the critically ill and their families on a daily basis in an environment which is fast-paced and where support systems are needed.

The effect of stress on one's health status and well-being should be noted. Creating a comfortable, humane physical environment, which is conducive to the individual's well-being, should have a high priority for nursing service and nursing education administrators. Lack of responsive nursing leadership and a stressful physical work environment were identified in the studies reviewed in this chapter as causative factors of stress of CCU Nurses.

New Directions for Research on Nursing Stress

As noted earlier, the primary focus of research on stress in nursing practice has been the identification and rank-ordering of psychologic stressors of Critical Care Nurses. However, reports of stressors of nurses in other areas of practice are beginning to emerge. For example, the following studies indicate new speciality areas in nursing which are currently being investigated: (1) studies of Hospice Nurses (Barstow, 1980; Garfield and Jenkins, 1980; Chiraboga, Jenkins and Bailey, in press); (2) a study of Oncology Nurses (Donovan, 1981); (3) an investigation of stress of Head Nurses (Leatt and Schneck, 1980); and (4) a study of stress of Operating Room Nurses (Preston, Ivancevich, and Matteson, 1981).

Although research on nursing stress is beginning to have an impact in developing awareness on the complex nature of nursing, new directions for research need to be considered. The following areas are suggested:

- Comparative studies of stressors of Critical Care Nurses with stressors of nurses in other areas of practice need to be conducted.
- Correlates of psychosocial stress with nursing behaviors such as absenteeism, medication errors, somatic complaints, and patient outcomes such as length of hospitalization and presence of complications associated with nursing care need to be investigated.
- Relationship between stress and organizational variables such as leadership style, centralized or decentralized structure, and management modality of nursing care, needs to be investigated.
- Stressors, coping strategies, and social support systems of top and middle nurse managers in both nursing education and nursing service need to be identified and compared.
- The effectiveness of Stress Management Programs conducted in nursing service at nursing education settings need to be systematically evaluated.

With the establishment of an expanded data base, nurse clinicians, nursing service directors, faculty, and nursing education administrators can begin to deal with the issue of nursing stress from an empirical perspective rather than from an approach which is intuitively based.

Chapter Summary

Since the mid-1960's, the psychologic stress of Critical Care Nurses has been an expanding area of inquiry. A computerized search and review of some 100 articles on stress of nurses led the authors to develop definitive criteria and a rationale for selecting a sample of studies on the stress of Critical Care Nurses for review and evaluation. Seven studies of psychologic stress of Critical Care Nurses met the criteria. Studies were reviewed, evaluated, and compared primarily on the basis of methodology and findings. Implications for nursing education and nursing service, and limitations of the studies were summarized. New directions for future research were suggested. Although the knowledge base for identifying stressors of Critical Care Nurses has recently expanded, there is a need for greater empiricism and for scientific study of additional stress-related factors in nursing.

REFERENCES

Aiken, L.H., Blendon, R.J. & Rogers, D.E. The shortage of hospital nurses: A new perspective. *American Journal of Nursing,* 1981, *81*(9), 1612-1618.

American Nurses' Association. *Inventory of registered nurses* 1977-78 Kansas City, Missouri: Author, 1981.

Anderson, C.A. & Basteyns, M. Stress and the critical care nurse reaffirmed. *Journal of Nursing Administration,* 1981, *11*(1) 31-34.

Appley, M.H. & Trumbull, R. On the concept of psychological stress. In *Psychological Stress, Issues in Research.* New York: Appleton-Century-Crofts, 1967.

Ashley, J.A. Power in structured misogyny: Implications for the politics in care. *Advances in Nursing Sciences,* 1980, *2*(3), 3-21.

Bailey, J.T. Stress and stress management: An overview. *Journal of Nursing Education,* 1980, *19*(6), 5-8.

Bailey, J.T. The critical incident technique in identifying behavioral criteria of professional nursing effectiveness. *Journal of Nursing Education,* 1980, *19*(6), 15-24.

Bailey, J.T., Steffen, S.M. & Grout, J.S. The stress audit: Identifying the stressors of ICU nursing. *Journal of Nursing Education,* 1980, *19*(6), 15-24.

Barstow, J. Stress variance in hospice nursing. *Nursing Outlook,* 1980, *28*(12), 751-754.

Cassem, N.H. & Hackett, T.P. Sources of tension for CCU nurse. *American Journal of Nursing,* 1972, *72*(8), 1426-1430.

Chiriboga, D., Jenkins, G., & Bailey, J.T. Stress and coping among hospice nurses: Test of analytic model. (In Press)

Claus, K.E. & Bailey, J.T. *Living with stress and promoting well-being.* St. Louis: C.V. Mosby Company, 1980.

Donovan, L. The shortage. *R.N.,* 1980, *43*(6), 21-28.

Donovan, M.I. Stress at work: Cancer nurses report. *Oncology Nursing Forum,* 1981, *8*(2), 22-25.

Eisdorfer, C. Critique of the stress and coping paradigm. In C. Eisdorfer (Ed.) *Models for clinical psychopathology.* New York: Medical and Scientific Books, 1981.

Facts About Nursing 80-81. New York: American Journal of Nursing Company, 1981.

Garbin, M. Stress and research in clinical settings. *Topics in Nursing,* 1979, *1,* 87-95.

Garfield, C., & Jenkins, G. Stress and coping of volunteer grief counselors. *Omega,* 1981.

Grout, J.W., Steffen, S.M. & Bailey, J.T. The stresses and the satisfiers of the intensive care unit: A survey. *Critical Care Quarterly,* 1981, *3*(4), 35-45.

Hay, D. & Oken, D. The psychological stress of intensive care unit. *Psychomatic Medicine,* 1972, *34,*(2), 109-117.

Huckabay, L. & Jagla, R. Nurses' stress factors in the intensive care unit. *Journal of Nursing Administration,* 1979, *9*(2), 21-26.

Jacobson, S.P. Stressful situations for neonatal intensive care nurses. *American Journal of Maternal Child Nursing,* 1978, *3*(3), 144-150.

Koumans, A.J.R. Psychiatric consultation in an intensive care unit. *Journal of the American Medical Association,* 1965, *191* (6), 163-167.

Lazarus, R.S. Cognitive and personality factors underlying threat and coping. In M.H. Appley & R. Turnbull (Eds.) *Conference on Psychological Stress.* New York: Appleton-Century-Crofts, 1967.

Leatt, R. & Schneck, R. Differences in stress perceived by head nurses across nursing specialities in hospitals. *Journal of Advanced Nursing,* 1980, *5,* 31-46.

Lewis, F.M. The nurse as lackey: A sociologic perspective. *Supervisor Nurse,* 1976, *7*(4), 24-27.

Mason, J.W. A historical view of the stress field, part II. *Journal of Human Stress,* 1975, *1,* 22-36.

Melton, C.E., McKensie, J.M., Polis, D.B., Hoffman, M. & Saldivar, J.R. *Physiological response in air traffic control personnel: Houston intercontinental tower.* (FAA AM 73-21) Washington: U.S. Office of Aviation Medicine, 1973.

Millar, S. Real issues behind the critical care nursing shortage. *Heart and Lung,* 1980, *9*(5), 801-802.

Miller, T.W. Life events scaling: Clinical methodological issues. *Nursing Research,* 1981, *30*(5), 316-320A.

Pelletier, K. *Mind as healer: Mind as slayer.* New York: Delacorte, 1977.

Polis, B.D., Polis, E., Decani, J., Schwarz, H.P., & Dreisbach, L. Effect of physical and psychic stress on phosphatidyl glycerol and related phospholipids. *Biochemical Medicine,* 1969, *2,* 286-312.

Polit, D.F. & Hungler, B.P. *Nursing research: Principles and methods.* Philadelphia: J.B. Lippincott Company, 1978.

STRESS AND CRITICAL CARE NURSING

Preston, C.A., Ivancevich, J.M. & Matteson, M.T. Stress and the OR nurse. *American Operating Room Nurses Journal*, 1981, 33(4), 662-671.

Robinson, A.M. ICU '72. The R.N.: Without her, no ICU's. *R.N.,* 1972, *35*(3), 46-51.

Selye, H. Confusion and controversy in the stress field. *Journal of Human Stress,* 1975, *1*(2), 37-44.

Selye, H. Stress and a holistic view of health for the nursing profession. In K.E. Claus & J.T. Bailey (Eds.) *Living with stress and promoting well-being.* St. Louis: C.V. Mosby, 1980.

Smith, D. Organization theory and the hospital. *Journal of Nursing Administration,* 1972, *2*(3), 19-24.

Steffen, S.M. Perceptions of stress: 1800 nurses tell their stories. In K.E. Claus & J.T. Bailey (Eds.) *Living with stress and promoting well-being.* St. Louis: C.V. Mosby, 1980.

Vreeland, R. & Ellis, G.L. Stresses on the nurse in an intensive care unit. *Journal of the American Medical Association,* 1969, *208*(2), 332-334.

Wandelt, M.A., Pierce, P.M., & Widdowson, R.R. Why nurses leave nursing and what can be done about it. *American Journal of Nursing,* 1981, *81*(1), 72-77.

Wolf, G.A. Nursing turnover: Some causes and solutions. *Nursing Outlook,* 1981, *29*(4), 233-236.

Chapter Seven:
Research Studies in
Hospital Staff Development

Chapter Seven:
Research Studies in
Hospital Staff Development

Mary O'Leary, R.N., M.H.P.Ed.
Bette Case, M.S.N.
Deborah Marks, M.P.H.

Introduction

This chapter reviews research and evaluation studies related to staff development in a hospital setting. Staff development is defined as that part of learning which the agency offers to increase the employees' knowledge and skills in relation to the role expectations within the agency. Staff development may include any or all of the following: orientation, skills training, management training and inservice education.

Continuing education has been excluded because its goals are different. It has a much broader scope and is characterized by educational offerings designed to present newly emerging concepts of health care, principles, theories and research in health care and nursing which enhance the professional knowledge base and enable nurses to practice at increasingly higher levels of excellence.

What questions are currently being asked by staff development investigators conducting research and evaluation studies in staff development in a service setting? Are questions being asked within a theoretical framework? What are their findings? Can the studies be replicated? How successful are the findings in revealing information that is applicable to a staff development department in a service setting? Are the findings significant and could they have an impact on the organization, program development and evaluation of future programs? What recommendations can be offered for further study in the field? The literature was reviewed with these questions in mind.

This review includes: variables studied; number of subjects; instruments used; and findings. Discussion and implications for future studies are included.

The literature was selected for review only when the author's conclusions were supported by data. There are many articles which describe programs but they have been eliminated from this review because they are not data based (Borovies and Newman, 1981; Giles, 1981; Holloran, 1982; Horn, 1981; Mersenhelder, 1982; Paparone, 1980; Pinkney-Atkinson, 1980; Plasse and Lederer, 1981). Articles which describe cost effective formulas or techniques were also eliminated (Boyer, 1981; Del Bueno and Kelly, 1980; Marenco, 1978; Rantz, 1980; Schmalenberg and Kramer, 1979; Sovie, 1980). Articles on guidelines for evaluating skills or programs were also eliminated from the review because they did not include actual research or evaluation studies (Hofing, McGugin and Merkel, 1979; Holzemer and Bridge, 1979; Kibbee, 1980; Kneedler, 1976; McMahon and Neuman, 1972; Michnich, Shortell and Richardson, 1981; Norman and Hoffman, 1976; Prescott, Jacox, Collar and Goodwin, 1981; Rufo, 1981). Finally, performance appraisal and quality assurance were eliminated from this review since each topic could become a separate review.

The literature review in staff development has been divided into three categories; these include Orientation Programs, Inservice Education Programs, and Participation in Staff Development Programs. Each section is reviewed.

Orientation Programs

Orientation programs have examined the following independent variables: type of orientation program (Peitchinis, 1978; Kramer and Schmalenberg, 1978; May, Minehan and Deluty, 1981); type of educational preparation (Peitchinis, 1978; Schroeder, Cantor and Kurth, 1981); previous experience (Peitchinis, 1978); and staffing pattern (Peitchinis, 1978). In addition, Roell (1981) identified characteristics of nurse internship programs and McCorkle, et al. (1979) evaluated a special orientation program designed to prepare nurses to function in an oncology unit.

Peitchinis (1978) examined the effect of three types of orientation programs on the performance of newly hired registered nurses. The three types of programs were: traditional orientation (N=20); ten-day precepted experience on an orientation unit (N=9); three-day precepted experience on an orientation unit (N=29). Clinical performance was assessed at five intervals during the first six months of employment with the Slater Nursing Competencies Rating Scale over the following five areas of nursing practice: psychosocial, (individual), psychosocial (group), physical, general communication, and professional. The total sample size was 58. She reported that nurses' competence increased gradually over their first six months of employment in all groups. Their 13- and 26- week scores were significantly higher than their four- and nine- week scores, which were significantly higher than their two- week ratings. Improvements were demonstrated in the total rating score and in all areas of the Slater Scale expect psychosocial (group).

The nurses in the study were graduates of three-year hospital, two-year hospital, and two-year college programs. Highest scores were obtained by the three-year hospital graduates and lowest by the two-year college graduates. The significant difference in the performance of the three educational groups was found beginning in the fourth week of their employment. No significant differences were found among graduates with no work experience. When the nurses were grouped according to their work staffing pattern, there were no significant differences in their performance.

The quality of patient care rendered by the nursing staff before and after the introduction of the two experimental orientation programs (ten-day and three-day) was assessed with Phaneuf's nursing audit of patient's chart and Wandelt's Quality Patient Care Scale (Qualpa CS). Measurements were taken on three occasions: before the introduction of the first orientation unit, seven months after its introduction, and nine months after the introduction of the second special unit. A random sample of six patients from each patient care unit was selected for the patient care assessment.

The Quality Patient Care Scale data revealed that there were significant differences in the quality of care rendered over a period of time. Nursing audit supported a difference in the quality of care provided on the basis of staffing patterns for application and execution of physician's legal orders, observations of symptoms and reactions, supervision of patient and total audit score. Comparisons

125

between the nurses' assessed competence and the quality of care observed suggested that in many instances, nurses' scores were higher than those assigned by observers to the nursing practice witnessed.

Schroeder, Cantor, and Kurth (1981) identified orientation learning needs on the basis of educational preparation. They used Cantor's Process-Oriented Goal-Directed Model to establish the content required for nursing practice. The learning needs of the nurse were identified in terms of patient needs. They constructed four measures to assess learning; these were the Emergency Test, the Medication Test, Complications Test and the Experience Checklist.

The study sample consisted on 146 new graduates with six months or less experience. Ninety-one were from baccalaureate programs (71 from the program associated with the study hospital); 36 were from diploma programs, 19 from associate degree programs. The tests were administered during the general orientation program. Pretests were scheduled to precede presentation of content by the orientation staff.

They found no major areas mastered by all graduates and the level of mastery varied widely. The scores did not differ appreciably by type of educational program. The findings revealed that there were no areas of content that could be eliminated from orientation for a particular group. They concluded that it was not possible to predict content needs on the basis of type of educational program. The data also suggested that these educational programs have not established criteria-based mastery levels for factual content needed for safe and effective nursing care. No group demonstrated complete mastery of the evaluation component of the nursing process.

Kramer and Schmalenberg (1978) reported on a nation-wide survey of inservice education departments in eight medical center hospitals. The purpose of the study was to determine if a special role transformation designed to foster biculturalism would ease new graduate nurses' adjustment to the work world and consequently decrease the exodus caused by the reality shock phenomenon. They developed a "Role Transformation Program" consisting of two orientation programs. One was a Clinical Training Program (CTP) which was similar to traditional hospital orientation programs and the second was the Bicultural Training Program (BTP). Both programs had the same format and length. The BTP focused on content needed to develop biculturalism and to effect a positive role transformation containing affective, cognitive and behavioral components. The affective component, Referent Group Development, started six weeks after employment and consisted of seminars designed to help new graduates deal with conflict in school and work on an emotional level. The cognitive component was called Path to Biculturalism and was designed to provide participants with the knowledge base necessary in mediating conflicting demands and value systems. The third component, Conflict Resolution, consisted of several all-day workshops for new graduates and head nurses.

The instruments used for the program evaluation were: Corwin's Role Conception Scale, "What Action Would You Take?" (measured respondents' reported role behavior in conflict situations), The Personal Orientation Inventory, Tennessee Self-Concept Scales, and Empathy (modification of Dymond tool). In addition, interviews of participants, head nurses and co-workers were conducted providing performance ratings. Employment status data were also collected. The sample was 307 new graduate nurses in their first nursing job in eight medical centers in the U.S.

After approximately one year of employment, data were collected. They found that professional role conception was significantly higher for nurses in the BTP as compared to the CTP. The bicultural role behavior choices of nurses in the BTP were higher than those of nurses in the CTP. The number of changes instituted and their effectiveness was higher for the BTP nurses than for the CTP nurses. Performance ratings of the nurses in the BTP were higher than those of nurses in the CTP. Employment status data collected one year after employment indicated that 90% of the biculturally trained nurses were still employed and 10% had resigned. Of the CTP nurses, 60% were still employed and 40% had resigned. It appeared that the BTP orientation program was effective in assisting new nurses to maintain professional role conceptions, choose bicultural role behaviors, institute effective changes, perform better, and remain in the organization longer.

May, Minehan and Deluty (1981) subsequently reported on an evaluation of bicultural training. Their hospital sponsored a leadership training program given by Kramer and Schmalenberg to prepare nurses to implement a bicultural role transformation program. Five nurses completed the program and 21 new graduates participated in portions of the program. The objectives were to increase the participants' length of tenure and to improve work performance of new graduates. Two instruments were used. One was the Professional Performance Evaluation Tool (PPET), a 75-item descriptive list of nursing behaviors. The second was an Acceptability Questionnaire, a 14-item questionnaire to elicit subjective responses from bicultural program participants in relation to specific issues: time/scheduling factors, program's influence on job satisfaction, perceived benefit to self, and change agent activity. Both were designed by the investigators. The sample was 41 new nurses. Twenty-one participated in the leadership training program (the experimental group) and 20 new graduate nurses hired during the same time period as those nurses in the experimental group but who had not participated in the leadership training program (control group).

There was no significant difference in tenure between the experimental and control groups (65% of the control group were still employed at the time of the data collection as compared to 57.1% of the experimental group). There were also no significant differences in mean performance evaluation scores between the two groups. The authors did not feel the results of their study could be generalized. They suggested that institutions using a system of nursing care other than primary nursing might see a more significant effect produced by the program.

Roell (1981) surveyed nurse intern programs throughout the country. A 31-item questionnaire examined four aspects of nurse internship programs: administrative, structural, content and clinical. The sample was 43 JCAH approved non-profit, non-federal hospitals having a bed capacity of 375 or more.

The reason programs were instituted was because new graduates and their supervisors believed new graduates were unable to function independently in the clinical area. The interns usually received less than full staff nurse salary during the program. Most internship programs were coordinated by staff development or in-service education. Most programs accepted four to 50 interns with a mean of 20. The programs ran from six weeks to one year with an average of 13 weeks. All of the programs offered annual and semi-annual intern programs. The content focused on knowledge and skills the new nurse needed to function in a staff nurse role and progress was monitored often through periodic written evaluations and weekly conferences. Formal classroom instruction averaged 6.5 hours per week. The content of formal classroom instruction was determined primarily by needs expressed by the interns. However, over half of the respondents stated that some classroom content was predetermined by inservice staff and head nurses on the basis of perceived deficiencies in the new nurses' basic nursing education programs. The respondents indicated that most interns received experience on multiple units with tours of all three shifts. Nearly all institutions used general medical-surgical units for rotations and a small number included specialty or critical care.

In 1979, McCorkle, Denton and Georgiadou evaluated the effectiveness of a three-week orientation class. The purpose of the orientation program was to prepare newly appointed staff to function in a new multidisciplinary cancer unit. Two instruments were used. A self-report assessed what the learner says about herself and what she has learned and was developed by the staff. Forty-six objectives based on six areas of knowledge and skills were included (cancer content related to specific disease, treatment protocols, and nursing interventions; management and leadership concepts; and group interaction and leadership skills).

The second questionnaire contained questions related to job expectations and satisfaction, nurse-doctor relationships, degree of distress of common problems, situations that cause stress, activities to relax and reduce stress, amount of support for job from other people and how important the goals of the unit are or should be.

The first instrument was distributed before the start (Time 1) and again at the close of the orientation class (Time 2). The second instrument was distributed two months after the unit had been fully operational (Time 3). The subjects were 28 female nurses with a variety of previous nursing experiences, ranging in age from 23-38 years. Ninety percent of the nurses had baccalaureate degrees.

Over 75% of the staff reported an increase in their knowledge and skills after the orientation program. Only 54% of the staff reported an increase in their overall knowledge and skills after having worked on the unit for nine weeks. In fact, 18% reported a lower score after working than they had identified on their pretest. The authors felt that one explanation for this may have been that the staff perceived themselves as having more knowledge than they actually had when placed in the clinical setting. However, only one content area (staging of disease) was rated lower. The other lower ratings were related to use of resources, management and leadership.

The orientation studies reviewed are descriptive in nature. The following dependent variables were measured: nursing knowledge, clinical behavior and/or perceptions of self in the work setting (Peitchinis, 1978; Kramer and Schmalenberg, 1978; May, et al., 1981; Schoeder, et al., 1981; McCorkle, et al., 1979) and quality of patient care (Peitchinis, 1978).

Inservice Education Programs

Review of the studies related to inservice education programs documents assessment of learning needs (Buechler, 1982; Kasprisin, et al., 1981; Grossbach-Landis and McLane, 1979); program evaluation (Merkel, et al., 1980; O'Leary and Holzemer, 1980; O'Leary, 1979; Vendura, 1979; Distefano and Pryer, 1975) and evaluation of teaching methods (Huckabay, et al., 1977). Data analyzed included performance on written examinations (Kasprisin, et al., 1981; Huckabay, et al., 1977; Distefano and Pryer, 1975); performance in simulated clinical situations (Buechler, 1982; O'Leary and Holzemer, 1980); performance in clinical situations (Grossbach-Landis and McLane, 1979) and clinical data (Buechler, 1982; Merkel, et al., 1980; O'Leary, 1979; Vendura, 1979).

Buechler (1982) evaluated mock resuscitation code drills in order to improve performance during a real emergency. A mock code rating scale which lists activities to be carried out during an arrest was used. Points were assigned to each activity according to how important the activity is in the effective, safe and organized handling of a code; i.e., three points were given to activities contributing directly to the maintenance of life, 0.5 points given to those activities that did not directly contribute to maintaining a patient's life in the manner identified. Eighty percent or above was to be considered a "passing grade".

Thirteen nursing care areas in a 410-bed acute care facility were used to carry out mock codes on all three shifts. The number of nurses participating in the mock codes was not given. Prior to conducting the mock arrests, inservice programs consisting of the viewing and discussion of a videotape on mock codes were conducted for all staff on a 24-hour basis.

Though ratings on the mock code rating scale were not reported, the author identified poor CPR skills and lack of leadership on the part of team leaders as major problem areas. The investigator made recommendations to administration concerning identifying roles and responsibilities of staff on the clinical units related to monitoring real arrests, equipment and the proficiency of CPR skills of staff. One year after the recommendations had been implemented, the mock drills were again conducted in the same manner. The results showed only five nursing care areas below the 80% passing mark. Of those five, no area was below 65%.

The investigator did not discuss whether or not other inservices regarding CPR skills and roles and responsibilities related to codes were offered to staff between the two mock drills or how the recommendations from the first trial had been implemented.

Grossbach-Landis and McLane (1979) identified the learning needs of registered nurses who suction intubated patients. A 21-item observation tool developed by one of the investigators was divided into five sections: equipment, sterile equipment, assessment, psychological support and procedure. The sample was 30 full-time R.N.'s, eight from the respiratory intensive care unit and 22 from the surgical ICU. Only registered nurses who regularly suctioned intubated patients were observed. These included seven associate degree graduates (Group I); 12 diploma graduates (Group II) and 11 baccalaureate degree graduates (Group III). Patients included in the study were those with oratracheal tubes, nasotracheal tubes, or tracheostomy tubes in place. No children under age seven were included in the study.

In the overall sample the mean score for proper equipment utilization was 97%; for maintenance of sterile environment, 91%; for patient assessment, 38%; for psychological support, 57%; and for procedure, 62%. The overall mean score was 65%. These findings did not relate meaningfully to the amount of inservice, level of preparation, or years of experience.

Kasprisin, Kasprisin, Marks, Yogore and Williams (1981) assessed the knowledge base of registered nurses regarding blood component therapy and blood administration in order to develop content for an educational program. The need for this study was established by members of the nursing staff at a university hospital who did not think their knowledge base of the subject was adequate and who were concerned with maintaining safe, quality patient care.

A 16-item examination was used to measure transfusion therapy expertise. Nine of the questions were designed to test the nurses' knowledge of how to administer blood and how to properly read and identify a blood bag label. The other questions were specific to specialty areas and were not discussed in the findings. Four questions were clinical simulations which asked the nurse to decide between various labels to determine the proper unit for administration. Labels from actual units of blood or components were used in six of the nine questions. The sample size was 74 registered nurses: 22 bachelor of science, 28 diploma graduates, 17 associate degree graduates, one master of science and 6 unknown. The amount of experience ranged from two months to 27 years with the mean equal to 6.6 years.

The findings of the study revealed that many nurses did not have adequate knowledge of blood transfusion therapy. The results of this study identified the need for both assessment of nurses' learning and the development of an educational program. An inservice program was recommended and later developed and jointly presented by the Blood Bank and the Staff Development Department.

The results of the testing revealed that few nurses carefully examine a blood bag label. One reason given by many nurses for not examining blood labels was their assumption that the blood bank never made mistakes. Many of the nurses stated they had never been formally taught how to read a blood bag label or to administer blood. The test also revealed that the nurses did not fully understand which blood types are compatible. The nurses did better answering practical questions regarding blood administration. The test results were not related to type of education or years of experience.

O'Leary and Holzemer (1980) reported a program evaluation conducted to measure the extent to which nurses who had been certified in a Venipuncture Certification program retained their venipuncture skills, through demonstration, two to eight months after successfully completing the program.

The instrument used to evaluate nurses' performance was a checklist. It was the same checklist which had been used in the Venipuncture Certification Program as a tool to certify the nurses. Development of evaluation criteria from procedural descriptions in the literature was done to insure content validity of the instrument. Nurses received two points for skills "Done Correctly," and a score of zero was given for skills done "Incompletely," "Incorrectly," or "Not Done." A total of 38 points could be scored for each performance evaluation.

Three groups of ten inpatient and ambulatory care nurses employed in a large medical center hospital were randomly chosen. Group A consisted of nurses who had completed the program requirements for certification and who would be evaluated on the basis of their skill in drawing blood from a patient. Nurses in Group B had completed the program requirements for certification and would be evaluated according to their skill with a simulated arm. Group C was comprised of nurses who had not participated in the program and who would be evaluated according to their skill with the simulated arm. To select nurses for Group A and B, names of the 106 participants who had successfully completed the program requirements were listed alphabetically and every fourth name on the list was alternately assigned to either Group A or B until there were ten nurses in each group.

In the first phase of the study, Group A performed venipuncture on a patient and Group B performed venipuncture on a simulated arm. The performance of each group was compared. No significant difference in the performance of each group was found and it was concluded that the use of the simulated arm was appropriate for measuring performance of venipuncture skill.

In the second phase of the evaluation the simulated arm was used to compare the performance of Group B with the performance of nurses who had not enrolled in the program, Group C. The difference between the scores of the two groups was found to be significant at the .01 level. Nurses who had completed the program had significantly higher scores than those who had not completed the program. In addition, 10 of the 14 nurses who had been certified (six from Group A and four from Group B) had acceptable scores above 36, whereas no nurses from Group C had an acceptable score.

The most important finding was that participants who completed the program retained and were able to demonstrate their skills two to eight months later. The study also demonstrated the viability of using a simulated arm for evaluating venipuncture skills and showed that nurses who had not participated in the program were unable to perform venipuncture successfully.

O'Leary (1979) evaluated the effects of an intravenous therapy course on specific complications associated with intravenous therapy. The design used in the study was the interrupted time-series design. A series of measurements were taken before and after the introduction of the treatment. The incidence of complications was examined between June 1976 and October 1978. The last training sessions were completed in June 1977. Frequency of complications for 119 consecutive weeks was used. For the purpose of the analysis the effects of the intervention were expected to manifest themselves after June 1977.

The study was conducted at a major medical center hospital and 48 nurses and 120 medical students attended the course. IV associated complication rates such as septicemia, IV site infection and phlebitis were collected by a team of infection surveillance nurses.

The results of the data analysis did not indicate any significant decrease in complication rates following the introduction of the IV Therapy Course. There were many factors which contributed to these results. Only 16 of the 48 nurses trained completed all certification requirements of the course. Many of the 120 medical students left the hospital to complete their clinical rotations in other hospitals.

There were no hospital-wide policies available to outline IV therapy procedures or to support the course. It is possible that the IV Therapy Course did not appear to effect the IV complication rates because the effects of such a course may only be evident after a much longer latency.

Vendura (1979) reported on the positive effects of a newly developed pharmacology course in lowering the number of recorded medication errors, in reducing education costs and in reallocating resources to patient care. Prior to implementation of this new program the hospital had offered a traditional in-service program for newly employed L.P.N.'s. The program was problematic for participants, educators and head nurses. In spite of the program a significant number of medication errors occurred. A new educational program was developed to promote competency in drug administration by requiring proof of drug knowledge and demonstration of skill in dispensing medication. The program was less time consuming and was competency based. It was directed to all newly hired licensed practical nurses, all newly hired graduate nurses and newly hired registered nurses who had been licensed less than one year or who had not been actively involved in acute care nursing for two years or more. In the first year of the program, 50 registered nurses and 20 L.P.N.'s participated in the program.

As a result of the new program there were dramatic effects on the cost of education. The 70 participants spent only 420 hours in the new program as compared to 2,520 which would have been required in the old program. However, no R.N.'s actually participated in the traditional program. Participation by R.N.'s (new graduates and inexperienced R.N.'s) was under consideration at the time the new program was implemented. Therefore, R.N. hours are projections and not actual hours spent in the traditional program.

In comparing cost (actual and projected) $4,773 was spent to educate the 70 participants in the new program whereas $14,688 would have been spent for the same number of people in the former program. Vendura states that $9,915 were reallocated to patient care.

Finally, there were fewer recorded medication errors during the first year of the program than in the previous 12 months. Reported errors by L.P.N.'s decreased from 31 to 14; by graduate nurses group from 78 to six; by R.N.'s group from 110 to 109. Because the only R.N. participants in the new program were those recently licensed or without recent nursing experience, few of the total R.N. population of the institution participated. Many more L.P.N.'s and graduate nurses participated in the program than did R.N.'s. A significant decrease in medication error rate was seen among those groups whose participation in the program was greatest.

Vendura cites great satisfaction with the competency based program on the part of participants, inservice educators and nursing staff. The dollar savings results are somewhat questionable since actual reallocation of education hours to patient care took place only in the L.P.N. group.

Distefano and Pryer (1975) evaluated the effect of a training program on mental health knowledge and attitudes of nurses and nurses' aides in a general hospital. They predicted that psychiatric nursing knowledge and mental health attitudes would improve in selected groups of nursing personnel as a result of a six-week training program.

Two instruments were used to assess changes in those participating in the program. One was a basic psychiatric knowledge test which consisted of 33 multiple choice items. The second was the Opinions and Mental Illness (OMI) scale to measure mental health opinions and attitudes.

Two groups of nursing personnel from a public general hospital participated in the training program. The first group of trainees consisted of 15 female nurses — 12 registered nurses and three licensed practical nurses. The second group of trainees consisted of 14 nurses' aides — 12 female, two males. A comparison or control group of 14 nurses' aides were matched with the training group on the basis of pretraining psychiatric knowledge test scores.

The results reported a significant improvement in both training groups on psychiatric nursing knowledge. No statistically significant change in mental health attitudes was found on the Opinions about Mental Illness (OMI) scale in the nurse group but a significant reduction in social restrictiveness was revealed in the nurses' aide group. No significant change in knowledge or attitudes was found in the matched group of nurses' aides.

The investigators suggested that the results of the research indicated that brief psychiatric training can increase the psychiatric nursing knowledge of both professional nurses and nurses' aides. The results also suggested that brief training can improve attitudes of nurses' aides toward mental illness. The aides were significantly less restrictive in their attitudes toward mentally ill patients after training.

Merkel, McGugin and Hofing (1980) evaluated an instructional program on problem oriented records. The educational program was based on the theory that learning is observed through cognitive, behavioral and attitudinal changes.

The instruments included a subjective evaluation of the leraning activities, pre- and posttests to measure changes in knowledge, attitude, and skill, and a chart audit to review the format of the nurses' charting on the unit.

Group I (N=28) were staff on six patient care units where POR had been implemented previously and Group II (N=32) were staff on three patient care units where POR had not been implemented. The learners were comprised of R.N.'s, L.P.N.'s and student nurses.

The same test was administered before and after the educational program. The means of the pretest/posttest scores for both groups significantly improved. A chart audit on seven charts in the ICU was conducted over a six-week period to measure changes in charting behavior. Although the audit reflected a marked improvement in the staff's ability to collect and record data, seven charts is not a sufficient sampling to firmly support this conclusion. Furthermore, it was not stated whether or not ICU nurses participated in the POR education program. However, the authors felt that the data clearly indicated that the POR educational program was effective in the areas of changing knowledge, skills and attitudes.

Huckabay, Cooper, and Neal (1977) examined the effects of different teaching techniques on cognitive learning and affective behavior of nurses participating in a class on the theory of loss. The subjects in the study included 131 staff nurses, team leaders, and charge nurses from 15 hospitals who were enrolled in an inservice education class. They worked in chronic or acute general hospitals and cared for medical-surgical patients who were experiencing loss. The subjects included graduates from diploma, associate degree and baccalaureate programs.

Subjects were divided into four treatment groups: The E group (N=36) was taught by means of filmstrip and discussion (FD). Control groups II, III, and IV (N=33, 31 and 31 subjects, respectively) were taught by means of lecture alone (L), lecture with discussion (LD) and filmstrip alone (F), respectively. Pre- and posttest measured cognitive learning. An affective measure assessed the subject's feelings about the program and the format of the presentation. The E group learned significantly more than the L group; in general all groups showed significant increases in learning and transfer; film groups transferred significantly more than the lecture groups; subjects preferred lecture with discussion and filmstrip with discussion significantly more than filmstrip or lecture.

Participation in Staff Development Programs

Mishra (1979) reported on a study conducted to assess registered nurses' opinions regarding the factors responsible for participation and non-participation in a formal inservice education program in a selected hospital in Orissa State (India). She examined factors which facilitate and inhibit participation. Seventy-two R.N.'s working as nurse-clinicians, nurse administrators and nurse educators in the hospital were surveyed. The results indicated that no opportunity for attending inservice programs had been made available for nursing personnel in the institution. The majority of the respondents had a strong interest in attending programs of this nature. However, this desire seemed to wane with the advancement of age, increased experience, less income and less educational background.

Matthews and Schumacher (1979) assessed the needs and participation factors for continuing education in nursing on the part of 150 R.N.'s in two hospital settings. Eighty-nine questionnaires were returned from nurses in a 1,100-bed university hospital and 61 from a 360-bed community hospital.

Fifty to seventy-five percent of the respondents characterized continuing education activities as being of relatively short duration, on specific topics and resulting in a certificate of completion or credit toward a higher academic or professional degree. Twenty-three percent or less thought continuing education activities should present several topics and last longer than one week. Eighty-eight percent of the respondents believed that continuing education activities are necessary to maintain professional competence. Benefits most frequently mentioned were increased knowledge and skill, increased awareness of current nursing trends, better patient care and maintenance of professional competence.

Ninety-six percent of the respondents thought credit or CEU's should be awarded for participation in continuing education activities. Only 48% thought mandatory continuing education should be required by law for nursing license renewal. Factors rank ordered as least important in considering participation in a continuing education activity were: 1) whether or not CEU's were given, 2) length of activity and 3) dollar cost. The most important participation factors included relatedness of topic to job, personal interest in a topic, perceived need or information and the time of the activity.

DelBueno (1977) reported on a two-part continuing education workshop conducted to provide an opportunity for inservice directors to design, implement and evaluate a research project in inservice education. Each project was to evaluate effectiveness and efficiency of an offering. During the first two-day session participants reviewed the steps in the research process, practiced writing objectives and differentiated between evaluation methods and measurement tools. They also completed an initial description of their project and determined the behavioral objectives for the inservice offering.

At the second two-day workshop 11 participants had completed all or some of the objectives for their projects and reported their results. Subject matter for the projects included: monitoring arterial blood pressure; writing nursing care plans; CPR; medication administration by L.P.N.'s; initiating and implementing a CPR team; management of a female patient with an indwelling catheter; and effectiveness of preoperative teaching.

The author felt that an important outcome of this workshop was that the inservice directors seemed to have changed their approach to resolving learning needs. Those who had implemented research projects recognized the importance of measuring effectiveness and efficiency of inservice activities. Participants identified their own learning needs in relation to research and evaluation. This journal article is reported not because it is a data-based research study, but because it illustrates efforts to implement research in staff development settings.

Conclusion

Questions investigated in staff development related to effects of different types of orientation programs, educational preparation of nurses, characteristics of internship programs, assessment of learning needs, program development, program evaluation, effects of different teaching techniques and patterns of participation. Few of the studies reviewed were based upon a theory. The studies have been summarized in the categories of orientation, inservice programs and participation patterns. The diversity of the findings prohibits further classification and summary. Problems in replication of several of the studies cited include: incomplete description of tools; use of convenience sampling rather than controlled sampling procedures; small sample size; insufficient information regarding data collection and analysis; and unsupported assumptions. For application of the findings, careful examination of the characteristics of one's institution is required to determine the degree of correspondence to the study setting.

These authors suggest that further research and evaluation may wish to focus upon theory building for staff development. Possible avenues appear to be theories of learning and theories of nursing and client care outcomes. Increased use of clinical performance and other clinical data as dependent variables is recommended. Study of management training programs is needed. Staff development educators should become more active in research and evaluation efforts. Contributions in these areas will facilitate evaluation and research based staff development practices.

REFERENCES
Borovies, D.L., and Newman, N.A. Graduate nurse transition program. *American Journal of Nursing,* October 1981, *81*(10), 1832-1835.

Boyer, C.M. Performance-based staff development: The cost-effective alternative. *Nurse Educator,* September-October 1981 *6*(5), 12-15.

RESEARCH STUDIES IN HOSPITAL STAFF DEVELOPMENT

Buechler, D. Code blue evaluation. *Nursing Management,* May 1982, *13*(5), 25-28.

Del Bueno, D. Evaluation of a continuing education workshop for inservice educators. *The Journal of Continuing Education in Nursing,* March-April 1977, *8*(2), 13-16.

Del Bueno, D.J., and Kelly, K.J. How cost-effective is your staff development program? *Journal of Nursing Administration,* April 1980, *10*(4), 31-36.

Distefano, M.K. and Pryer, M.W. Effect of brief training on mental health knowledge and attitudes of nurses and nurses' aides in a general hospital. *Nursing Research,* January-February 1975, *24*(1), 40-42.

Giles, E.L. New nurse program lowers turnover. *Hospitals,* August 1981, *55*(16), 60-61.

Grossbach-Landis, I., and McLane, A. Tracheal suctioning: A tool for evaluation and learning needs assessment. *Nursing Research,* July-August 1977, *28*(4), 237-242.

Hofing, A.L., McGugin, M.B., Merkel, S.I. The importance of maintenance in implementing change: An experience with problem-oriented recording. *The Journal of Nursing Administration,* December 1979, *9*(12), 43-48.

Holloran, S.D. Teaching male catheterization: An application of change theory for an entire nursing staff. *Nurse Educator,* January-February 1982, *7*(1), 11-14.

Holzemer, W.L., and Bridge, T.L. Guidelines for evaluating hospital-based continuing education programs. *Quality Review Bulletin,* August 1979, *2*(7), 2-7.

Horn, R. Planning inservice education in small hospitals. *Supervisor Nurse,* January 1981, *12*(1), 38-41.

Huckabay, L.M., Cooper, P.G., and Neal, M.C. Effect of specific teaching techniques on cognitive learning, transfer of learning, and affective behavior of nurses in an inservice education setting. *Nursing Research,* September-October 1977, *26*(5), 380-385.

Kasprisin, C.A., Kasprisin, D.O., Marks, D., Yogore, M.G., and Williams, H.L. Quality assurance beyond the bloodbank. *Supervisor Nurse,* May 1981, *12*(5), 45-48.

Kibbee, P. Developing a model for implementation of an evaluation component in an orientation program. *The Journal of Continuing Education in Nursing,* September-October 1980 *11*(5), 25-29.

Kneedler, J. Criterion referenced measurement for one continuing education offering: Pre and postoperative visits by operating room nurses. *The Journal of Continuing Education in Nursing,* March-April 1976, *7*(2), 26-36.

Kramer M., and Schmalenberg, C. Bicultural training and new graduate role transformation. *Nursing Digest,* 1978, *5*(4), 1-47.

Marenco, E. Accounting concepts and techniques for managing continuing education and inservice. *Nursing Administration Quarterly,* Fall 1978, *3*(1), 75-80.

Matthews, A.E. and Schumacher, S. A survey of registered nurses' conceptions of participation factors in professional continuing education. *The Journal of Continuing Education in Nursing,* January-February 1979, *10*(1), 21-27.

May, L., Minehan, P., and Debuty, L. Evaluating bicultural training. *Journal of Nursing Administration,* May 1981, *11*(5), 24-29.

McCorkle R., Denton, T., and Georgiadou, F. Evaluation of a program for a cancer unit. *Cancer Nursing,* August 1979, *2*(4), 274-276.

McMahon, J., and Neuman, M.M. Tool for evaluating the impact of an inservice program on nursing care. *The Journal of Continuing Education in Nursing,* March-April 1972, *3*(2), 5-7.

Meisenhelder, J.B. A first-hand view of the unit teacher role. *Nurse Educator,* March-April 1982, *7*(2), 17-20.

Merkel, S.I., McGugin, M.B., and Hofing A.L. Evaluation: The often neglected aspect of POR education. *Supervisor Nurse,* October 1980, *11*(10), 68-71.

Michnich, M.E., Shortell, S.M., and Richardson, W.C. Program evaluation: Resource for decision making. *Health Care Management Review,* Summer 1981, *6*(3), 25-35.

Mishra, R. Factors influencing participation and non-participation in a formal inservice education program for nursing personnel in a state government hospital in Orissa. *The Nursing Journal of India,* March 1979, *LXX*(3), 71-75.

Norman, A.E. and Hoffman, K.I. The benefits of direct performance tests. *The Journal of Continuing Education in Nursing,* May-June 1976, *7*(3), 34-37.

O'Leary M.M. *Effects of an intravenous therapy certification course on IV complications.* Unpublished master's thesis, University of Illinois at the Medical Center, 1979.

O'Leary, M.M., and Holzemer, W.L. Evaluation of an inservice program. *Journal of Nursing Administration,* March 1980, *10*(3), 21-23.

Paparone, P. Developing a framework for inservice. *Supervisor Nurse,* October 1980, *11*(10), 29-30.

Peitchinis, J. Orientation programs and the competent nurse. *Dimensions in Health Service,* June 1978, *55*(4), 12-13.

Pinkney-Atkinson, V.J. Mastery learning model for an inservice nurse training program for the care of hypertensive patients. *The Journal of Continuing Education in Nursing,* March-April 1980, *11*(2), 27-31.

Plasse, N.J. and Lederer, J.R Preceptors — a resource for new nurses. *Supervisor Nurse,* June 1981, *12*(6), 35-41.

Prescott, P.A., Jacox, A., Collar, M., and Goodwin, L. The nurse practitioner rating form part I: Conceptual development and potential uses. *Nursing Research,* July-August 1981, *30*(4), 223-228.

Rantz, M.J. A modular approach to unit orientation. *Supervisor Nurse,* June 1980, *11*(6), 48-51.

Roell, S.M. Nurse-intern programs: How they're working. *Nurse Educator,* November 1981, *6*(6), 29-31.

RESEARCH STUDIES IN HOSPITAL STAFF DEVELOPMENT

Rufo, K.L. Guidelines for inservice education for registered nurses. *The Journal of Continuing Education in Nursing,* January-February 1981, *12*(1), 26-33.

Schmalenberg, C., and Kramer, M. Bicultural training: A cost effective program. *Journal of Nursing Administration,* December 1979, *9*(12), 10-16.

Schroeder, D.M., Cantor, M.M., and Kurth, S.W. Learning needs of the new graduate entering hospital nursing. *Nurse Educator,* November 1981, *6*(6), 10-17.

Sovie, M.D. The role of staff development in hospital cost control. *The Journal of Nursing Administration,* November 1980, *10*(11), 38-42.

Vendura, N. Pharmacology program produces results. *Journal of Nursing Administration,* September 1979, *9*(9), 34-39.

Chapter Eight:
The Clinical Nurse Specialist

Chapter Eight:
The Clinical Nurse Specialist

Patricia Sparacino

The role of the Clinical Nurse Specialist (CNS) is one which will ultimately affect the state of the art of clinical nursing practice. The CNS can be the most appropriate means by which nursing practice is knowledgeably and accurately investigated and new nursing knowledge is introduced. Likewise, the role of the CNS can influence the advancement of nursing in a more clinical direction by requiring that direct patient care, when appropriate, be provided by registered nurses, in contrast to the managerial practice of nursing where patient care is provided by staff other than registered nurses (Christman, 1973, p. 39). Because the CNS considers "various alternatives in making assessments and prescribing nursing actions...[she] consciously utilizes inductive and deductive reasoning to organize data so that nursing decisions are precise and relevant to the problem under investigation" (Niessner, 1979, p. 23). Hence, clinical specialization, by applying scientific reasoning to the nursing care of patients, will expand the extent of nursing practice. If the ultimate effect a CNS has on nursing practice were comparable to that of a medical specialist on medical practice, then the "efficiency ratio" of nurses' impact on patient care outcomes could be raised considerably (Christman, 1973).

HISTORICAL PERSPECTIVE   The concept of the nurse as a specialist was first described by DeWitt in 1900, with the designation given to those nurses who had graduated from specialized hospitals or private-duty nurses who limited their practice to the care of particular types of patients. By the 1950's a specialist was a nurse who was recognized to have developed a high level of skill as well as knowledge in a particular area of nursing practice. In 1961, Frances Reiter proposed the role of a "nurse clinician" or CNS who, because of her advanced clinical knowledge and expertise in clinical practice, would improve nursing care by means of a scientific approach to patient care. Reiter's concept of a CNS would demonstrate and provide nursing care, plan and supervise patient care given by other nurses, and serve as staff consultant and educator. In the 1960's it became generally recognized that a CNS was not only a designation for an expert clinician but that graduate preparation in a specified area of clinical nursing was an essential requisite. At the same time the number of clinical nurse specialists was becoming sufficient to begin to have an increasing impact on the health care delivery system. Yet, despite this increasing agreement as to appropriate preparation for the CNS, questions were still being raised as to the expected capabilities of the CNS in regard to role functions, interdisciplinary relationships, and innovative possibilities for the improvement of patient care (Little, 1967). In 1980, the American Nurses' Association defined the CNS as a nurse who, through preparation and practice at the master's or doctorate level, has become a recognized expert in a specified clinical area of nursing. The disagreement as to functional role components and administrative implementation persists.

EDUCATIONAL PREPARATION   The first master's degree program for clinical specialization was developed by Hildegarde Peplau at Rutgers—The State University of New Jersey in 1954. The program was in advanced psychiatric nursing, rather than the functional areas of education or administration which had preceded that of clinical specialization. Today, it is recommended that graduate preparation of the CNS place emphasis on the study of multidimensional components of health and illness and the development of expertise in a defined area of clinical practice. A major emphasis in the graduate program must be the development of a broad theoretical base of knowledge upon which to assess health care needs, predict patient behavior, plan and implement individualized nursing interventions, and evaluate patient outcomes on an advanced level (Dirschel, 1976).

FUNCTIONAL ROLE COMPONENTS Problems have existed with the evolution and utilization of the CNS role. Usually these problems can be attributed to misuse, underutilization, or abuse. The CNS has variously "functioned" as an expert clinician, nurse practitioner, head nurse, supervisor, combined head nurse-supervisor, associate director of nursing, nurse liaison, consultant, role model, change agent, educator for patients and staff, and researcher. With the evolution of the role there has been disagreement among nurse specialists themselves as to what the role responsibilities are. Confusion arises as to when a nurse is a specialist and when a nurse's functional capabilities have been expanded to assume tasks formerly carried out by the physician (Cahill, 1973). This confusion about the CNS role definition is often due to individualized role definitions. Nursing staff compare the variability among clinicians regarding actualization of their roles, and confusion about the similarities and dissimilarities between specialists emerges (Disch, 1978; MacPhail, 1971). Likewise, when the prevailing expectations of high-level people in the professional system range from the ideal and unattainable to total aberration, the effective functioning of the CNS will be impeded.

As the CNS role has evolved, it is agreed that the four functional role components are those of patient care, consultation, education, and research. The CNS, as an expert clinician, assesses the patient with a high level of discriminative judgment, determines priorities of care, designs, with advanced knowledge and skill, and implements comprehensive, individualized quality patient care. This continuity of care assists patients, complementing their capacity to achieve or maintain optimum health and functioning (Armacost, 1973; Backsheider, 1971; Dirschel, 1976; Simms, 1965). The CNS must not only demonstrate technical and humanistic expertise in providing direct patient care but must manifest innovative or creative nursing practice. The CNS as expert clinician goes beyond the use of intuition or generalizations, calling for a scientific accountability for professional attitudes and nursing practice. The clinical nurse specialist's expertise likewise provides a practical relevance when developing a theoretical framework for nursing practice (Niessner, 1979). The clinical nurse specialist's involvement in patient care ranges from her working collaboratively with members of the health care team to taking a patient assignment or carrying a specific case load and working alone. When working independently, the care the patient received from a CNS will be excellent, but the nursing staff will not benefit from cooperative interaction with the CNS and will not, therefore, function any differently in relation to the care of their patients; nor will nurses assuming a clinical nurse specialist's patient's care be prepared to adopt those aspects of care for which the CNS had been responsible (Crabtree, 1979).

As a consultant, the CNS is available to members of the health care team and participates with them in a process of problem-solving based on theoretical knowledge and clinical expertise. By assisting nurses to clarify a problem situation, the nurses will learn to achieve patient care goals more efficiently and to develop the ability to solve a wider range of nursing problems (Armacost, 1973; Dirschel, 1976). The CNS consultant is not a part of any particular administrative group, but rather works in an institution-wide staff position. If perceived as a "threat" or as an evaluator by nursing staff, they may subsequently be reluctant to refer patients to the CNS or to implement suggestions. Therefore, to be truly effective, she must be an experienced clinician with leadership ability, communication skills, and administrative backing (Barrett, 1972; Blake, 1977).

The CNS as educator serves the needs of patient, family, staff nurse and members of the health care team. The CNS's role in patient and family education goes beyond that which the staff nurse is able to provide, specifically patients who, due to their unique physical condition or heightened anxiety, have special learning needs. The CNS's effect on the quality of patient care delivered is achieved by improving the educational preparation of all nurses, thereby theoretically influencing the quality of care for all patients. By providing education to satisfy the growth needs of all levels of nurses, the CNS builds a strong staff. In this manner she acts as a stimulus to improve the overall quality of patient care. Frequently the CNS can assist staff to more quickly attain their learning goals by simplifying learning needs, compiling information from the literature, and providing inservice education. When instructing staff at the patient's bedside, the role modeling effect can dramatically assist staff to increase their clinical competencies (Armacost, 1973; Dirschel, 1976; Everson, 1981; Smith, 1974).

The research component of the CNS role can be varied in its implementation, but the effect is the same, that of improving the quality of nursing care by means of scientific inquiry and the application of the research process to clinical and theoretical nursing problems (Dirschel, 1976). While clinical nurse specialists already critique published research to evaluate and implement what is applicable to the practice setting, too few clinical nurse specialists are actively involved in nursing research. Only in this way will a scientific basis for nursing practice be expanded (Jacox, 1974).

Whether seen as an integral component of the CNS role or as a fifth and separate component, it is generally agreed that the CNS is a role model and change agent. While modeling *per se* is an admirable but difficult goal to achieve, the CNS is nonetheless capable of disseminating expert knowledge and demonstrating resourcefulness. Furthermore, a spirit of inquiry, ready adaptability, a predilection for research and the ability to establish effective nurse-physician collaboration in achieving exemplary patient care are essential aspects to ensuring the success of the role in the practice setting (MacPhail, 1971).

THE ROLE OPERATIONALIZED One of the areas of greatest disagreement in the effective utilization of the CNS role is the placement of the CNS in the nursing hierarchical system. The CNS role is an administrative anomaly which does not comfortably fit into the bureaucratic management system of a health care institution (Niessner, 1979; Parkis, 1974; Stevens, 1976). Confusion about CNS role implementation revolves around the primary issues of professional versus administrative authority. Professional authority evolves as a result of knowledge and expertise and should, theoretically, apply to every competent CNS. Administrative authority is granted to the position, by virtue of the job description and placement within the organization, rather than extrinsically to the individual (Stevens, 1976).

The CNS, with administrative or line authority, generally assumes the role of head nurse, supervisor, or associate director of nursing. Several authors (Barrett, 1972; Castronovo, 1975; Johnson, 1967) concur that the advantage a CNS has in a line position is the necessary authority to enforce clinical decisions, evaluate patient care and experiment with alternate approaches in improving the comprehensiveness and quality of patient care. The administrative authority makes available the reward power to hold staff accountable and to invoke sanctions necessary when staff are noncompliant in heeding recommendations. The line position gives the responsibility and authority to the CNS to work within the existing organization and to ultimately effect change (Edwards, 1971; Niessner, 1979; Odello, 1973).

The way in which a CNS utilizes the line position has been variously implemented. Most often discussed in the literature is the CNS as nursing supervisor. Crabtree (1979) advocates the use of the CNS as a clinical nursing supervisor who would be accountable for patient care as well as personnel, while the head nurse would assume responsibility for administrative tasks. The CNS would then serve as a consultant for management problems but as an evaluator of the implementation of the nursing process. Fagin (1967) and Butts (1974) view the role of supervisor as expanded to include clinical specialization. This encompasses a concept of an authority role effecting change, as well as the CNS serving as staff developer, an evaluative overseeing role which assists the staff nurse to develop clinical skills. This approach to role implementation is supported by the cost control factor that would make more available the number of people who could theoretically function both as supervisors and as clinical nurse specialists.

Beeber and Scicchitani (1980) prescribe that the CNS's most expeditious as well as effective means of improving the delivery of patient care is by becoming a part of the nursing team so that, by working through nursing care problems together with staff nurses, a CNS can understand the operational problems of administering patient care. The rationale for placing the CNS in a unit-based structure is that it is otherwise demoralizing to the nursing staff to witness a CNS prescribe nursing care or arrive at a solution to a problem with apparently no appreciation for the overall demands of the unit. When the CNS demonstrates expertise in improving patient care while coping with the number of non-related demands encountered, then she will be accepted by staff.

When the CNS is in a line position, it is extremely difficult for her to apportion time to management needs as well as clinical responsibilities. Therefore, the administrative demands of the position will divide the clinical nurse specialist's energies to the detriment of clinical responsibilities and thus limit time allocated for direct patient care (Parkis, 1974; Stevens, 1976). Besides limitations on clinical involvement, other disadvantages of the CNS in a line position are that the CNS may not have had graduate preparation in nursing administration and, if the CNS also serves as staff evaluator, there may be staff reluctance to ask for the clinical nurse specialist's assistance in theory or skill acquisition, fearing a show of ignorance will reduce the possibility for acknowledgment within the institution (Beeber and Scicchitani, 1980; Crabtree, 1979).

Beeber and Scicchitani (1980) describe the CNS in a staff position as a multidimensional functional model who directly improves patient care by delivering expert care, and who indirectly improves patient care by interacting with staff nurses, other clinical nurse specialists, members of the health care team, and institutional administrators in the areas of education, consultation, and research. When the CNS is in a staff position she is freed from administrative non-nursing tasks. Her power is derived from expert power, expert knowledge, clinical competency and referent power, as well as her personality characteristics. She is able to maintain a consultative relationship with the consultee who is more apt to ask for assistance than if the CNS were in a line position (Beeber and Scicchitani, 1980; Everson, 1981; Jackson, 1973).

The disadvantage of the CNS in a staff position is that she must build and withstand the testing of her professional authority, frequently a slower route than assuming the given administrative power of a line position. The utilization of the CNS will depend upon staff understanding of the role and role functions and their perception of patient needs (Crabtree, 1979; Stevens, 1976). With no formal authority over the implementation of patient care, CNS frustration can be high and accountability limited. Therefore, it has been difficult to measure the effect of the CNS on the quality of patient care delivered or on patient outcomes when her access to patients is dependent upon the perception of need and referral by others (Stevens, 1976).

Role ambiguity evolves when there is no clear pre-existing consensus of CNS role expectations. A common job description with room for individualization would minimize this ambiguity by defining where within the organizational plan the CNS is placed, to whom she is directly responsible, the type of authority with which the position is empowered, and the qualifications that must be brought to the position.

PROBLEMS ENCOUNTERED IN THE CNS ROLE   One of the problems in discussing the role of the CNS is that the specialist classification does not automatically assume a person's clinical expertise in a specified area of nursing. Clinical expertise must be proven through practice, and it must be an integral part of the remaining functions of consultant, educator, and research. No component of the role can be deemed unimportant by a person professing to be classified as a CNS; nonetheless, there has been an ongoing relegation of scientific inquiry via research to a low, if not non-existent, priority.

The issue of collaborative efforts between the CNS and staff nurse can affect not only patient care but the effectiveness of the CNS role. Ehrenreich and Stewart (1979) state that:

> While the line position encompasses administrative or supervisory functions, the position designation does not in itself ensure that the specialist's recommendations regarding an individual's nursing care will be followed by the nursing staff. It will accomplish no more than the staff position designation will. (p. 263).

Subsequently the CNS experiences frustration when a decision about a change in patient care implementation is made by someone other than herself and which conflicts with her original recommendation. Therefore, if the fundamental goal of the CNS is better patient care, it would seem that the ultimate resolution would be not one of administrative authority or expert or referent power, but one of functional authority, as a physician has, in the directing, ordering, and giving of patient care (Armacost, 1973; Backsheider, 1971; Crabtree, 1979; Ehrenreich and Stewart, 1979).

The introduction of the CNS position into an existing hierarchical structure is a particularly difficult one when the CNS is presented with the problem of simultaneous role development and role implementation. Role ambiguity also evolves when there is no clear consensus of role expectations, especially when the CNS, hospital administrators, and staff nurses do not share similar expectations. Such a situation will only lead to frustration and role ineffectiveness, ultimately diminishing staff nurse perception of the value of the CNS role. Even if the CNS has a clear understanding of the role and how it should be implemented, the most important precursor to success is administration's recognition of, and hence sanction of, the value of the role and its effect on quality patient care (Backsheider, 1971; Baker and Kramer, 1970: Castronovo, 1975; Colerick, Mason and Proulx, 1980).

RESEARCH REVIEW   Research on the role of the CNS has been in process since the mid-1960's, with a majority of published research appearing in the late sixties and early seventies. Little has been published since, and most has been descriptive. The topics of research have described attitudes toward the role of the CNS, CNS effect on nursing practice and patient outcomes, as well as how the role is operationalized, and problems encountered.

Miller's (1965) early descriptive study examined the characteristics of graduate nursing students being prepared as expert clinicians, teachers and supervisors. Sixty-one graduate students at one program were tested using the Strong Vocational Interest Blank for Women (SVIB), the California Psychological Inventory (CPI), two brief questionnaires measuring attitudes toward nursing and problems faced in nursing, and a one-hour interview designed to give life-history information. Data analysis differentiated among the four clinical specialties (medical-surgical, maternal-child, psychiatric, public health).

Findings of the SVIB demonstrated a positive correlation between the nurse scale and occupational scales most characteristic of the medical-surgical, maternal-child, and public health groups, while there was a negative correlation for the psychiatric group. In the CPI, the psychiatric group ranked highest on the tolerance psychological-mindedness scale. The psychiatric and maternal-child group differed most in personality; the medical-surgical group was similar to the psychiatric group and the public health was similar to the maternal-child group. The psychiatric group scored the highest in independence and the maternal-child group scored highest in self-insight. This type of research may be important when considering comparisons of different CNS roles as the role differences may be due to pre-existing differences, not role expectations.

HOW THE CNS ROLE IS PERCEIVED   Boucher and Bruce (1972) and Smith (1972) address the activities of clinical nurse specialists. While Boucher and Bruce directly address the perception of roles of the CNS by various health care providers and the value on certain CNS functions, Smith describes perceptions of functions of clinical nurse specialists as well as three other categories of nursing personnel. Each study was exploratory, utilizing questionnaires to allow participants to describe individual perceptions of role applications and how certain functions within each role were valued.

Using a 3-part questionnaire, with items derived from the literature, Boucher and Bruce sampled 24 nursing educators from two collegiate schools of nursing, and 12 clinical nurse specialists, 53 nursing administrators, and 47 nursing practitioners from ten general hospitals in a metropolitan area. The study's purpose was to assess the acceptance of the CNS role and the functions ascribed to it. Educators, clinical nurse specialists, and nursing administrators agreed in their perceptions of the CNS as an educator and researcher with practitioner expertise, but with little involvement as a change agent. The nurse practitioner differed in perceiving the role of the CNS as an educator and researcher with change agent competencies, but with little involvement with research or as an expert clinician. In their valuation of the CNS role, educators and nursing administrators appraised the CNS as an educator and practitioner with research competencies, but with little involvement with change planning or implementation. The CNS also valued the role as educator and practitioner, but valued their change agent competencies more than those functions which require research knowledge and skills.

Smith's descriptive study used a questionnaire, derived from Aradine and Denyes (1972), to categorize the judgment of six clinical nurse specialists, twelve head nurses, three nursing educators, and nine nursing service office personnel from a 460-bed hospital as to the appropriateness of 124 activity items in the areas of patient care, staff development, education, consultation, research, counseling, mobility, and administration. The activity items were also rank ordered by percentages of activities perceived to be performed from within categories as compared with performance across all categories. The significant finding of the study was the reflection of noncongruent expectations of role fulfillment between the CNS and the employing agency. Discrepancies were demonstrated between categories regarding CNS functions in relation to staff development, education, and patient care. Head nurses viewed clinical nurse specialists predominantly as consultants, while clinical nurse specialists perceived their primary role functions as not only consultants but as researchers as well. The CNS activity of practitioner in relation to patient care was ranked third by head nurses, but fourth by clinical nurse specialists themselves. Ultimately, however, there was little unanimity in any of the four categories about their own activities or activities of the other categories.

CNS EFFECT ON NURSING PRACTICE   To indirectly examine the issue of improving patient care, the effect of the CNS on nursing staff or nursing practice has been described. Georgopoulos and Christman attempted to overcome the problem of noncongruent role expectations and introduced the clinical nurse specialist position into three medical wards of a large teaching hospital. In 1970, they described their research project in progress. The study hoped to demonstrate that patient care units led by clinical nurse specialists would provide qualitatively and quantitatively superior nursing care as compared to those units continuing in the traditional mode. Two aspects of this study were subsequently reported by Georgopoulos and Jackson (1970) and Georgopoulos and Sana (1971).

The Georgopoulos and Christman research design introduced the clinical nurse specialist role into three 25-bed medical units, while three comparable control units were managed by traditional head nurses. While the experiment lasted for thirteen months, data were collected at three intervals. Data consisted of interviews with patients and various health care team members, recorded intershift reports, individual patient kardexes and various logs, observation forms, a nursing activity study, and special assessment instruments.

Georgopoulos and Jackson (1970) reported on the effectiveness of the CNS role as determined by patterns of nursing behavior data recorded on 764 patient kardexes. Comparisons of kardexes and of kardex data patterns on the experimental and control units were made during the thirteen month period, with particular emphasis on the difference between the beginning and end of the study. In order to classify and code kardex information and to code all substantive nursing statements, a research instrument was developed. The categories of substantive data were processed by two coders who then jointly discussed statements which were considered ambiguous. Overall intercoder agreement was 79%, or a reliability of .89. With independent recoding of ambiguous items, overall agreement rose to 86%.

In the quantity and distribution of substantive information, the patient care units led by clinical nurse specialists were more complete in coverage and demonstrated an increase in instrumental nursing functions, while the units led by traditional head nurses emphasized expressive nursing functions. In the quantity and distribution of evaluative information, both the experimental and control groups improved in five of the same care categories, but each group improved in two different categories. Without comparing the similarities and differences in the care categories and evaluative statements between the two groups, the experimental groups demonstrated a more clinical or patient-focused approach, with increasing improvement over time, while the control groups were more managerial or staff-focused in approach. The investigators felt that the data supported their hypothesis that nursing practice is measurably superior when influenced by the leadership of a CNS.

Georgopoulos and Sana (1971) then reported on the influence of clinical nurse specialists on the qualitative-evaluative nursing information given in intershift reports. Taken at three time intervals during the thirteen months of the study, 160 reports which covered 3,499 patients were analyzed. An instrument was developed which allowed coding the type of patient care, whether care was nurse-dependent or physician-dependent. The content of the intershift reports was analyzed by two master's-prepared nurses, with an intercoder agreement of 84%. Their results corresponded with those of the Georgopoulos and Jackson kardex study, particularly demonstrating an inverse relationship between groups and the evaluative statements which emphasize managerial and clinical concerns. By the third measurement of the study, the intershift reports of the control groups emphasized predominantly nursing managerial concerns, while the experimental groups' intershift reports stressed clinical patient care concerns, leading the investigators to conclude that the influence of the clinical nurse specialist at the patient care level can specifically affect intershift report behavior and generally affect nursing practice.

With similar intent, Ayers, Padilla, Baker and Crary (1971) introduced the clinical nurse specialist role at a teaching hospital to provide expert nursing care to a select group of patients. Initially the CNS was part of the nursing team and served as a team leader, but after six months and a new CNS, the role was changed to that of a resource person for a 57-bed medical chest unit. The CNS retained patient care responsibilities as well as serving as teacher and consultant. After nine months on the patient unit, a two-part study was developed to identify a unit's major nursing problems, systematically describe the integration of the CNS with staff and patients and compare the experience and acceptance, albeit effect, of three clinical nurse specialists with varying degrees of experience on three units.

The first stage of the study entailed the development of the Nursing Problems Priority Inventory (NPPI) which would ultimately test the effect of a CNS on the clinical insight of the nursing staff with whom she worked. To measure clinical insight, nurse-respondent was given two clinical situations for each of Abdellah's 21 nursing problems, with the degree of clinical competency determined by how many concrete clinical examples she/he could give for each situation. In determining inter-rater reliability of the NPPI, a one-way analysis of variance of a matrix of scores yielded 80% reliability. In testing the 42 NPPI items on 52 staff nurses, split-half reliability testing was done, and although 10 out of 21 reliability coefficients were significant at the .05 level, item reliability was not conclusively proven. The investigators agreed that although some test validity was indicated by the inter-rater reliability, the test was not yet fully developed and it was uncertain as to what it was that the test was actually attempting to measure.

The purpose of the second stage of the Ayers, et al. study was to measure the effect of the CNS on the nursing staff of the unit, and to describe the process by which a CNS developed within the role and related it to the nursing staff of a unit. The NPPI was administered to the staff nurses three times over a twelve-month period, with scoring measuring degree of increase in clinical insight. In addition, taped interviews with the clinical nurse specialists in the study, staff nurses, doctors and personnel from the experimental units were analyzed.

In comparing the three experimental and three control units, the control units showed overall the least increase in clinical insight. Among the experimental units, the unit which had an inexperienced CNS on an inexperienced unit showed the least increase in clinical insight. Although clinical nurse specialists were more accepted as time progressed, they had to deal with a lot of ambiguity in their roles and responsibilities; ambiguity was specified as being related to status, task, effect and career. An evaluation of the second stage revealed that the cognitive and emotional elements of the phases of CNS role development were those of orientation, frustration, implementation and reassessment with one CNS perceiving the four phases as being cyclic. There was agreement that a clinical nurse specialist's authority should concern clinical nursing issues, not administrative problems.

CNS EFFECT ON PATIENT OUTCOMES The largest number of studies on clinical specialization have occurred in the functional area of patient care. The first published results were those of Little and Carnevali (1967) who conducted an exploratory study to determine variations in patient response when care was given by a group of clinical nurse specialists. The subjects were 147 control and 164 experimental patients who had been hospitalized in a 400-bed county sanatorium for pulmonary tuberculosis, and the nurses were master's-prepared psychiatric clinical nurse specialists. Three study phases, each six months long, examined the effect of patient-centeredness nursing behaviors on patient response to illness. Nurse responses were obtained by tape recorded nurse-patient interactions collected at random hours of the day and week in the second and fifth to sixth month of each six-month phase. "Patient centeredness" was categorized using Matthews' categories and value system, and statistical comparisons between nurses and wards were made by a t-test of means. Patient response to illness was measured by physiological and behavioral data. Monthly statistical analysis was made of comparable inter-ward patient data as well as intra-ward comparisons. Analysis was by cohort analysis, with significance of differences preliminarily tested by chi-square, and finally analyzed by the t-test of means.

The major findings in the analysis of nursing behaviors were that the CNS spent more time in direct patient care, exchange of information, teaching and conferencing with staff about patient care, and that CNS behaviors influenced her professional and non-professional co-workers on the experimental ward. The outcomes of patients' responses to care given by clinical nurse specialists on the experimental ward was evidenced by radiological improvement, non-significant bacteriological results and longer duration of hospital stay, less involvement in self-care and a greater number of deviant behaviors and disciplinary transfers. Ultimately, therefore, patient responses, or improvement in radiological and bacteriologic results, length of hospital stay, involvement in self-care, and deviant behaviors, did not correlate with care delivered by psychiatric clinical nurse specialists.

Another study which assessed the effect of nursing care given by a CNS was by Murphy (1971). The subjects were 50 adult patients who were admitted to a university medical center and who were to undergo open-heart surgery by the same cardiac surgeon. The patients were graded as to severity of illness and were randomly assigned to three nursing care groups. The three nursing care groups: 1) received pre- and post-operative care by the CNS in addition to the customary care given by the staff nurses, 2) received post-operative care by the CNS in addition to the customary pre- and post-operative care by the staff nurses, and 3) received the customary care given by the staff nurses. Information gathered on the patients included assessment by the attending cardiac surgeon on the operative day through fifth post-operative day of the number and degree of any of the eleven most common post-operative complications, developed on a Likert scale; a daily assessment from recovery progress, scored as "yes" or "no" on a check list of activities; a 20-item Likert-type scale to evaluate the patients' perceptions and evaluations of hospital and nursing care; and relevant socioeconomic data.

The data were subjected to the chi-square method for determining independence of variables as well as searched for directional tendencies, but neither hypothesis could be supported. Therefore, the data were examined for descriptive information. Due to the negative findings, the investigators did not share the descriptive findings other than to say that the most common post-operative complications are body temperature alterations and cardiac arrhythmias, and that none of the 50 patients was assessed as having five or more post-operative complications.

Pozen, et al. (1977) studied 102 sequential myocardial infarction patients who consented to participate. The patients were randomly assigned to the study and control groups. The rehabilitation CNS met with the study group patients while in the coronary care unit, during their hospital convalescence, and by phone after hospital discharge. The questionnaires included an IPAT Anxiety Scale, the Hopkins self-report symptom inventory (HSCL-90), an objective knowledge questionnaire based on American Heart Association pamphlets and a self-report questionnaire. Analysis of the data demonstrated that the effect of the CNS rehabilitation supplementing patient care resulted in increasing patients' return to work and decreasing smoking, both significant at the .05 level. The study group patients also tested as having an increased knowledge of heart disease, significant at the .01 level. The CNS did not have an effect in reducing anxiety.

In a study built on the principle of the CNS improving nurse-dependent patient responses, Girouard (1978) examined whether the availability of a CNS would influence nurses to do more preoperative teaching. Two medical-surgical units in a general hospital were randomly assigned to be the experimental and control units, and a convenience sample of 36 nurses and 80 patients on the two units were studied. A pretest-posttest experimental design was used, with both groups of nurses and patients studied as to opinions and performance as related to pre-operative teaching. Information collected included opinions of staff about pre-operative teaching, and the incidence and kardex documentation of the pre-operative teaching. Prior to the CNS intervening with the experimental group, there was no significant difference, using t-tests, in opinion, activity, or actual pre-operative teaching performance. When the groups were given the posttest after the CNS intervention, there was no difference between groups in opinion nor claims about doing pre-operative teaching and documentation. However, the experimental groups did demonstrate a change in actual performance, significantly ($p < 0.004$) providing more pre-operative teaching and providing more documentation about the pre-operative teaching in the kardex ($p < 0.001$). Neither group demonstrated a significant increase in the amount of patient teaching documented in the nursing notes.

In a study specifically designed to compare the teaching effectiveness of clinical nurse specialists versus non-master's prepared nurses, Linde and Janz (1979) examined the effect of a structured comprehensive teaching program on knowledge and compliance in 48 patients who had had cardiac surgery in a large midwestern medical center. Twenty-five patients were taught by two master's prepared clinical nurse specialists and 23 patients were taught by four non-master's prepared staff nurses. Both patient groups received a pre-operative knowledge pretest before beginning the teaching program, and follow-up tests at the time of discharge from the hospital, and at the one-month and three-to-four-month post-operative outpatient visits. The structured comprehensive teaching program consisted of five to six sessions of 20-25 minutes each, covering the disease process and surgical intervention, activity progression, medication and dietary regimes, and risk factor modification. The only differences between the way the groups were treated was the educational preparation of the nurse educators and that the post-operative outpatient visit testing and teaching was done by the clinical nurse specialists.

The major instrument was a knowledge test which examined the major content areas of the teaching program, as well as specific questions for the valve replacement and coronary artery bypass patients. Except at the time of hospital discharge, the patients were tested at each interval about their medications. At each of the post-operative visits they were also tested for compliance by self-reporting on reduction of risk factors, laboratory follow-up, diet adherence, and attendance at clinic appointments. Content validity for the tests was established, but validity and reliability compliance on risk factors and diet modification were limited due to patient self-reporting.

The most significant finding was that the patients taught by the clinical nurse specialists had significantly (p < .002) higher knowledge test scores at discharge than the patients taught by the non-master's prepared staff nurses. Another significant finding was that not only did all the patients increase their knowledge test scores after receiving the post-operative patient education program, but there were no significant declines in test scores at the one-month or three-to-four-month post-operative visits.

PROBLEMS ENCOUNTERED BY THE CNS   The aspect of the CNS role that has been investigated the most is the description of problems encountered by the CNS when actualizing the role. When Baker and Kramer (1970) interviewed 22 directors of nursing in medical centers in the United States, the three areas which lent themselves to investigation were title designation, role functions and authority, and accountability of the CNS. The survey revealed that title designations are numerous, more often selected to satisfy a financing board than to clarify expectations from the role. In questioning the directors of nursing about CNS role functions, there was consensus that the goal was to improve patient care, but views were varied and divergent as to the activities of the CNS. All of the directors of nursing were concerned about the line versus staff placement of the CNS in the organizational hierarchy, to whom the CNS directly reported, and defined authority.

Another area of concern when attempting to actualize the CNS role is attitude of physicians toward the role. Barrett (1971) introduced the role of CNS, a practitioner with administrative responsibilities for nursing care, onto two separate 15-bed units in the surgical division of a university hospital. She then surveyed the surgeon's reactions to the role. She found that the surgeons felt that the high quality of patient care was directly attributed to the presence of the CNS, and likewise they felt that patient care was better when the CNS was responsible for the nursing care administration. Similarly, Davidson, et al. (1978) surveyed 200 psychiatrists to explore their attitude toward the role of the psychiatric nurse therapist (PNT), a master's-prepared psychiatric nurse clinician. A three-part questionnaire was designed to test the respondents' knowledge of the role, their willingness to utilize the role and their prior contact with a PNT, as well as demographic data. Knowledge, utilization and attitude scores were based on an assigned point system, with chi-square and chi-square significance levels calculated for each of the seven hypotheses. Correlation techniques of Spearman, Rank and Pearson's coefficient, as well as their significance levels, were performed on four of the hypotheses. Results from the data revealed that psychiatrists' attitudes about the PNT were positively correlated with the knowledge of and prior contact with a PNT. Also, those psychiatrists who rated themselves as having a higher degree of adherence to the psychoanalytic framework tended to score high for utilization of the PNT role.

Another problem which has hampered the understanding and full utilization of the role has been the broad scope of activities and pressures encountered. Aradine and Denyes (1972) reported the findings from a two-day symposium held specifically to explore the scope as well as developmental sequence of the activities and pressures of clinical nurse specialists. As a result of large and small group discussion, composite lists identified 122 activities and 59 pressures which were categorized into 12 activities and 4 pressures. Each participant then used the list to report her own degree of involvement and types of experiences over each of five time periods. The degree of involvement was tabulated by a scored point system. The Pearson-R correlation analyzed the activity-pressure interactions.

Some of the significant findings revealed that only 57% of the clinical nurse specialists were responsible for nursing care activities, with the remaining appointments being in the areas of joint clinical-faculty (21%), clinical and administrative (11%), and miscellaneous joint (11%). Sixty-one percent held line positions. Eighty-two percent were primarily unit-based, with the remainder serving by consultation. Categories of involvement in role activities usually reflected anticipated growth and development, with patient care being a major involvement initially. Involvement in activities broadened over subsequent time periods, but the categories of research, writing for publication and administration consistently showed a small degree of involvement.

Consistent with the scope of responsibilities is the issue of what factors influence job satisfaction for the CNS. Shaefer (1973) sampled 208 clinical nurse specialists, prepared at least at the master's level, and who were employed by hospitals greater than 200-bed capacity and associated with university medical centers. The data were collected by means of two questionnaires based on one developed by Lyman Porter to measure perceived need deficiencies in managers. The most significant finding was the negative relationship between perceived administrative support and CNS job dissatisfaction, significant at the .01 level. There was no relationship between the length of the master's program or salary received and job dissatisfaction. Also, the results of the study were not able to support previous studies which suggested a curvilinear relationship between length of a person's career and job satisfaction.

Finally, a similar study by Ehrenreich and Stewart (1979) questioned 194 clinical nurse specialists, employed in Veterans Administration hospitals affiliated with university medical schools, to determine whether there were commonalities in clinical nurse specialists' perceptions about their role. The organizational factors which were perceived by clinical nurse specialists as being facilitators or inhibitors were authority, changing of staff, rotating staff, advanced scheduling of hours and autonomy. A CNS in a line position, with administrative and supervisory functions, appeared to have no greater insurance of implementing clinical recommendations than did a CNS with a staff designation. Constantly changing staff, whether it was medical or nursing, decreased functional interactions due to the need for constantly establishing new relationships and interpreting the CNS role. Rotation of nursing staff among the three shifts also inhibited the accomplishment of goals. The clinical nurse specialists perceived the requirement to work advance-scheduled eight-hour-day shifts as interfering with accessibility to patients and families, availability for emergencies and flexibility in providing staff inservice education. Other inhibiting factors were lack of autonomy and reporting to a superior in an educational department.

Summary

The perception of activities and the role of the CNS are variously interpreted, often dependent simply upon whether the person being questioned has ever worked with a CNS. Boucher and Bruce (1972) discovered that a number of educators had never worked with or only briefly worked with a CNS, and a number of nursing administrators had only worked with a CNS indirectly. Although the literature described the CNS as a master clinician, none of Boucher and Bruce's respondents perceived clinical practice as an area of primary involvement for the CNS. Perhaps a resolution for this confusion would be the development of a CNS statement of performance expectations with precise behaviors describing CNS activities (Smith, 1974).

The desired outcome of the clinical nurse specialist's effect on nursing practice would be the CNS and staff nurse working collaboratively to improve the quality of patient care and patient outcomes as well as advance the state of nursing practice. More often, however, the CNS and staff nurse tend to function separately, resulting in little change in nursing practice. Woodrow and Bell (1971) felt that this discontinuity is due to three problems: 1) lack of mutual responsibility among nursing administration, nursing educators and clinical nurse specialists in defining how the goal of the clinical nurse specialist's effect on improving patient care is to be met; 2) staff nurses are not committed to involvement in the process, perhaps due to the CNS having no legitimate authority and therefore being unable to reward those nurses who emulate CNS role modeling; and 3) the CNS role is perceived as a threat by nursing staff. However, when a CNS is perceived as a clinical expert and has a leadership position and either a designated or acquired authority base which are visible, familiar and acceptable to staff and the CNS alike, then the CNS, as demonstrated in studies, will be able to positively affect nursing practice and patient care outcomes (Little and Carnevali, 1967; Georgopoulos and Jackson, 1970; Georgopoulos and Sana, 1971; Ayers, et al., 1971; Murphy and Schmitz, 1971; Pozen, et al., 1977; Girouard, 1978; Linde and Janz, 1979).

The issue of CNS authority is one of the many challenges or problems a CNS encounters. Ehrenreich and Stewart (1979) concluded that it is not so much an issue of possessing a line or staff position, as it is having a position of functional authority. Additional ingredients for predicted success of the CNS role are a clearly defined position statement of CNS activities, a title which is consistent with the functions expected, and organizational sanction of CNS authority to make change where and when appropriate (Baker and Kramer, 1970; Colerick, Mason and Proulx, 1980).

LIMITATIONS   Most of the research on the CNS role and its activities has been exploratory or descriptive, with little utilization of control groups. Only a few studies encompassed more than one site, and often the sample sizes were small.

This chapter reviewed five studies on CNS effect on patient care outcomes; and only three (Murphy, 1971; Pozen, et al., 1977; Linde and Janz, 1979) utilized a CNS whose clinical specialty was the same as the patients being studied. Little and Carnevali (1967) used psychiatric clinical specialists to provide physiological improvements in patients with tuberculosis, and Girouard (1978) did not identify the clinical specialty of the CNS employed. Future studies should always utilize a CNS with the same clinical specialty as the patients she is caring for if the CNS effect on patient care outcomes is to be studied with any validity.

Until there is consensus in the definition of the role of the CNS and its statement of practice, the direction of research studies will be uncertain. Clinical nurse specialists will need to come to an agreement as to precise behaviors describing CNS activities, how those behaviors affect nursing care, and their effect on psychological and/or physiological outcomes in the patient. Patient outcomes cannot truly be tested until a firm theoretical foundation is established for CNS practice.

GUIDELINES FOR AREAS OF FUTURE RESEARCH   Most of the literature which describes the role or its implementation is merely anecdotal accounts of activities and responsibilities, with very little of the literature consisting of research on particular aspects of the CNS role and its effect on nursing practice or patient care. Philosophies are expounded and idealisms are expressed, but more research is urgently needed to go beyond generalizations which do not have the benefit of experimental hypothesis testing.

It is the professional obligation of the CNS to conduct research which produces evidence of professional accountability and which contributes to the scientific basis of nursing practice. Listed below are just some of the numerous ideas for future research which have been suggested:

THE CNS ROLE
- A study of CNS activities which distinguishes the CNS role from a staff nurse role (Aradine, 1972).
- A study of the qualitative contributions of the CNS (Johnson, Wilcox and Moidel, 1967).
- Development of an instrument to document activities and pressures experienced over time (Aradine, 1972).
- A test of the effectiveness of different types of roles assumed by the CNS, i.e., CNS as patient care provider, CNS as supervisor, etc. (Georgopoulos and Jackson, 1970; Parkis, 1974).
- A study to determine the most effective basis of influence and degree of authority (Padilla and Padilla, 1979).
- A study of the effect of the variables of authority and power, albeit line versus staff, on the functioning of the CNS role (Ayers, 1971).
- A test of the model of the CNS as a practitioner but with administrative power to effectively change nursing practice (Padilla and Padilla, 1979).
- Development of a nursing theory base of CNS practice (Padilla and Padilla, 1979).
- A study of the relationship between what a CNS says she does and what she is actually doing.
- A study of when and why physicians refer patients to the CNS and what they expect the CNS to accomplish.

THE CNS AND PATIENT CARE
- A study of how CNS practice determines improved patient outcomes (Piazza, 1978).

- Development of an instrument to measure the amount of CNS versus staff time and effort expenditure to achieve desired patient outcomes (Aradine, 1972).
- A measurement of the quality of expertness of clinical judgments by the CNS (Christman, 1973).

THE EFFECT OF THE CNS ON HEALTH CARE ECONOMICS

- A study of the actual cost of the CNS in providing direct care to patients.
- A study of the relationship between improved patient outcomes and the number of litigations brought to bear (Piazza, 1978).
- A study of the relationship between CNS and staff nurse effect on decreasing the number of patient hospital days as well as decreasing patient recidivism.
- A study of the effect on patient care costs of collaborative practices of physicians and clinical nurse specialists.
- A study of the effect of CNS role modeling on staff nurse job satisfaction, improved patient service, and reduced attrition (Walton, 1973).

REFERENCES

Aradine, C. & Deynes, M.J. Activities and pressures of clinical nurse specialists. *Nursing Research,* 1972, *21*(5), 411-418.

Armacost, B. On becoming a nurse-manager of psychiatry. In J. Riehl & J. McVay (Eds.), *The clinical nurse specialist: Interpretations.* New York: Appleton-Century-Crofts, 1973.

Ayers, R., Padilla, G.V., Baker, V.E. & Crary, W.G. *The clinical nurse specialist: An experiment in role effectiveness and role development.* Duarte, California: City of Hope National Medical Center, 1971.

Backsheider, J. The clinical nursing specialist as a practitioner. *Nursing Forum,* 1971, *10*(4), 359-377.

Baker, C. & Kramer, M. To define or not to define: The role of the clinical specialist. *Nursing Forum,* 1970, *9*(1), 41-55.

Barrett, J. Administrative factors in development of new nursing practice roles. *Journal of Nursing Administration,* 1971, *1*(4), 25-29.

Barrett, J. The nurse specialist practitioner: A study. *Nursing Outlook,* 1972, *20*(8), 524-527.

Beeber, L. & Scicchitani, B. Should the clinical nurse specialist be free of administrative responsibility? *Perspectives in Psychiatric Care,* 1980, *18*(6), 250-269.

Blake, P. The clinical specialist as nurse consultant. *Journal of Nursing Administration,* 1977, *7*(10), 33-36.

Boucher, R. *Similarities and differences in the perception of the role of the clinical specialist.* Kansas City: American Nurses' Association's 8th Nursing Research Conference, 1972, Volume I.

Bruce, S. *Valuation of functions of the role of the clinical nursing specialist.* Kansas City: American Nurses' Association's 8th Nursing Research Conference, 1972, Volume II.

Butts, P. The clinical specialist vs. the clinical supervisor. *Supervisor Nurse,* 1974, *5*(4), 38-44.

THE CLINICAL NURSE SPECIALIST

Cahill, I. The development of maternity nursing as a specialty. In J. Riehl & J . McVay (Eds.), *The clinical nurse specialist: Interpretations.* New York: Appleton-Century-Crofts, 1973.

Castronovo, F. The effective use of the clinical specialist. *Supervisor Nurse,* 1975, *6*(5), 48-56.

Christman, L. The influence of specialization on the nursing profession. In J. Riehl & J. McVay (Eds.), *The clinical nurse specialist: Interpretations.* New York: Appleton-Century-Crofts, 1973.

Christman, L. The nurse clinical specialist. In J. Riehl & J. McVay (eds.), *The clinical nurse specialist: Interpretations.* New York: Appleton-Century-Crofts, 1973.

Colerick, E.J., Mason, P. & Proulx, J. Evaluation of the clinical nurse specialist role: Development and implementation of a dual purpose framework. *Nursing Leadership,* 1980, *3*(3), 26-34.

Crabtree, M. Effective utilization of clinical specialists within the organizational structure of hospital nursing service. *Nursing Administration Quarterly,* 1979, pp. 1-11.

Dambacher, E., Kirby, W., Masuda, M., Holmes, T.H. & Hoffman, K. Critique of the study: Nurse specialist effect on tuberculosis. *Nursing Research,* 1967, *16*(4), 327-332.

Davidson, K., et al. A descriptive study of the attitudes of psychiatrists toward the new role of the nurse therapist. *Journal of Psychiatric Nursing and Mental Health Services,* 1978, *16*(11), 24-28.

DeWitt, K. Specialties in nursing. *American Journal of Nursing,* 1900, *1*(1), 14-17.

Dilworth, A. Joint preparation for clinical nurse specialists. *Nursing Outlook,* 1970, *18*(9), 22-25.

Dirschel, K. The conception, gestation and delivery of the clinical nursing specialist. In R. Rotkovich (Ed.), *Quality patient care and the role of the clinical nursing specialist.* New York: John Wiley and Sons, 1976.

Disch, J. The clinical specialist in a large peer group. *Journal of Nursing Administration,* 1978, *8*(12), 17-20.

Edwards, J. Clinical specialists are not effective — why? *Supervisor Nurse,* 1971, *2*(8), 38-41, 45, 47, 51.

Ehrenreich, D. & Stewart, P. Clinical nurse specialists' perceptions of role facilitators and inhibitors in the practice setting. *American Nurses' Association Divisions of Practice: Clinical and scientific sessions.* Kansas City, Mo.: American Nurse's Association, 1979.

Everson, S. Integration of the role of clinical specialist. *The Journal of Continuing Education in Nursing,* 1981, *12*(2), 16-19.

Fagin, C. The clinical specialist as supervisor. *Nursing Outlook,* 1967, *15*(1), 34-36.

Georgopoulos, B. & Christman, L. The clinical nurse specialist: A role model. *American Journal of Nursing,* 1970, *70*(5), 1030-1039.

Georgopoulos, B. & Jackson, M. Nursing kardex behavior in an experimental study of patient units with and without clinical nurse specialists. *Nursing Research,* 1970, *19*(3), 196-218.

156

Georgopoulos, B. & Sana, J . Clinical nursing specialization and intershift report behavior. *American Journal of Nursing,* 1971, *71*(3), 538-545.

Girouard, S. The role of the clinical specialist as change agent: An experiment in preoperative teaching. *International Journal of Nursing Studies,* 1978, *15*(2), 57-65.

Jackson, B. Hospital administrators need to know about clinical specialists. *Supervisor Nurse,* 1973, *4*(9), 29-34.

Jacox, A. Nursing research and the clinician. *Nursing Outlook,* 1974, *22*(6), 382-385.

Johnson, D., Wilcox, J. & Moidel, H. The clinical nurse specialist as a practitioner. *American Journal of Nursing,* 1967, *67*(11), 2298-2303.

Knable, J. & Petre, G. Resistance to role implementation. *Supervisor Nurse,* 1979, *10*(2), 31-34.

Linde, B. & Janz, N. Effect of a teaching program on knowledge and compliance of cardiac patients. *Nursing Research,* 1979, *28*(5), 282-286.

Little, D. The nurse specialist. *American Journal of Nursing,* 1967, *67*(3), 552-556.

Little, D. & Carnevali, D. Nurse specialist effect on tuberculosis. *Nursing Research,* 1967, *16*(4), 321-326.

MacPhail, J. Reasonable expectations of the nurse clinician. *Journal of Nursing Administration,* 1971, *1*(5), 16-18.

Miller, D. Characteristics of graduate students in four clinical nursing specialties. *Nursing Research,* 1965, *14,* 106-113.

Morris, K. & Schweiger, J. Clinical nurse specialist role creation: An achievable goal. *Nursing Administration Quarterly,* 1979, *4*(1), 67-75.

Murphy, J. If p (additional nursing care): Then q (quality of patient welfare)? In M. Batey (Ed), *Communicating Nursing Research.* Boulder, Co.: Western Interstate Commission for Higher Education, 1971, *4,* 1-12.

Niessner, P. The clinical specialist's contribution to quality nursing care. *Nursing Leadership,* 1979, *2*(1), 21-30.

Nursing: A social policy statement. Kansas City, Mo.: American Nurses' Association, 1980.

Odello, E. The clinical specialist in a line position. *Supervisor Nurse,* 1973, *4*(9), 36-41.

Padilla, G. & Padilla, G. Nursing roles to improve patient care. *Nursing Digest,* 1979, *6*(4), 1-13. *53,* 29-31.

Padilla, G. & Padila, G. Nursing roles to improve patient care. *Nursing Digest,* 1979, *6*(4), 1-13.

Parkis, E. The management role of the clinical specialist. *Supervisor Nurse,* 1974, *5*(9), 44-51. (Part 1)

Parkis, E. The management role of the clinical specialist. *Supervisor Nurse,* 1974, *5*(10), 44-51. (Part 2)

Piazza, D. & Jackson, B. Clinical nurse specialists: Issues, power, and freedom. *Supervisor Nurse,* 1978, *9*(12), 47-51.

Pozen, M.W., Stechmiller, J.A., Harris, W., Smith, S., Fried, D.D. & Voight, G.C. A nurse rehabilitator's impact on patients with myocardial infarction. *Medical Care,* 1977, *15*(10), 830-837.

Reiter, F. Improvement of nursing practice. In J. Riehl & J. McVay (Eds.), *The clinical nurse specialist: Interpretations.* New York: Appleton-Century-Crofts, 1973.

Rogers, C. Conceptual models as guides to clinical nursing specialization. *The Journal of Nursing Education,* 1973, *12*(4), 2-6.

Shaefer, J. The satisfied clinician: Administrative support makes the difference. *Journal of Nursing Administration,* 1973, *3*(4), 17-20.

Simms, L. The clinical nursing specialist: An experiment. *Nursing Outlook,* 1965, *13*(8), 26-28.

Smith, M. The clinical specialist: Her role in staff development. *Journal of Nursing Administration,* 1971, *1*(1), 33-36.

Smith, M. Perceptions of head nurses, clinical nurse specialists, nursing educators, and nursing office personnel regarding performance of selected nursing activities. *Nursing Research,* 1974, *23*(6), 505-511.

ᵔmoyak, S. Specialization in nursing: From then to now. *Nursing Outlook,* 1976, *24*(11), 676-681.

Stevens, B. Accountability of the clinical specialist: An administrator's viewpoint. *Journal of Nursing Administration,* 1976, *6*(2), 30-32.

Walton, M. Professionals: Cost and quantity. *Nursing Clinics of North America,* 1973, *8*(4), 635-689.

Woodrow, M. & Bell, J. Clinical specialization: Conflict between reality and theory. *Journal of Nursing Administration,* 1971, *1*(6), 23-28.